T0320479

# Contemporary Applications of Mobile Computing in Healthcare Settings

R. Rajkumar
*VIT University, India*

A volume in the Advances in
Healthcare Information Systems
and Administration (AHISA) Book
Series

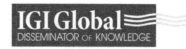

Published in the United States of America by
    IGI Global
    Medical Information Science Reference (an imprint of IGI Global)
    701 E. Chocolate Avenue
    Hershey PA, USA 17033
    Tel: 717-533-8845
    Fax: 717-533-8661
    E-mail: cust@igi-global.com
    Web site: http://www.igi-global.com

Library of Congress Cataloging-in-Publication Data

Names: Rajkumar, R. (Rajasekaran), 1976- editor.
Title: Contemporary applications of mobile computing in healthcare settings /
   R. Rajkumar, editor.
Description: Hershey PA : Medical Information Science Reference, [2018]
Identifiers: LCCN 2017033657| ISBN 9781522550365 (hardcover) | ISBN
   9781522550372 (ebook)
Subjects: | MESH: Mobile Applications | Telemedicine--instrumentation |
   Telemetry
Classification: LCC R855.3 | NLM W 26.55.S6 | DDC 610.285--dc23 LC record available at
https://lccn.loc.gov/2017033657

This book is published in the IGI Global book series Advances in Healthcare Information Systems and Administration (AHISA) (ISSN: 2328-1243; eISSN: 2328-126X)

British Cataloguing in Publication Data
A Cataloguing in Publication record for this book is available from the British Library.

All work contributed to this book is new, previously-unpublished material.
The views expressed in this book are those of the authors, but not necessarily of the publisher.

For electronic access to this publication, please contact: eresources@igi-global.com.

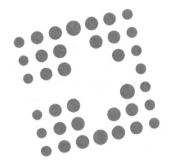

# Advances in Healthcare Information Systems and Administration (AHISA) Book Series

ISSN:2328-1243
EISSN:2328-126X

Editor-in-Chief: Anastasius Moumtzoglou, Hellenic Society for Quality & Safety in Healthcare and P. & A. Kyriakou Children's Hospital, Greece

## MISSION

The **Advances in Healthcare Information Systems and Administration (AHISA) Book Series** aims to provide a channel for international researchers to progress the field of study on technology and its implications on healthcare and health information systems. With the growing focus on healthcare and the importance of enhancing this industry to tend to the expanding population, the book series seeks to accelerate the awareness of technological advancements of health information systems and expand awareness and implementation.

Driven by advancing technologies and their clinical applications, the emerging field of health information systems and informatics is still searching for coherent directing frameworks to advance health care and clinical practices and research. Conducting research in these areas is both promising and challenging due to a host of factors, including rapidly evolving technologies and their application complexity. At the same time, organizational issues, including technology adoption, diffusion and acceptance as well as cost benefits and cost effectiveness of advancing health information systems and informatics applications as innovative forms of investment in healthcare are gaining attention as well. **AHISA** addresses these concepts and critical issues.

## COVERAGE

- IT Applications in Health Organizations and Practices
- Clinical Decision Support Design, Development and Implementation
- Nursing Expert Systems
- Telemedicine
- Role of informatics specialists
- E-Health and M-Health
- Virtual health technologies
- IT security and privacy issues
- IT Applications in Physical Therapeutic Treatments
- Management of Emerging Health Care Technologies

IGI Global is currently accepting manuscripts for publication within this series. To submit a proposal for a volume in this series, please contact our Acquisition Editors at Acquisitions@igi-global.com or visit: http://www.igi-global.com/publish/.

# Titles in this Series

*For a list of additional titles in this series, please visit:*
*https://www.igi-global.com/book-series/advances-healthcare-information-systems-administration/37156*

*Big Data Management and the Internet of Things for Improved Health Systems*
Brojo Kishore Mishra (C. V. Raman College of Engineering, India) and Raghvendra Kumar (LNCT Group of Colleges,India)
Medical Information Science Reference ●©2018 ● 312pp ● H/C (ISBN: 9781522552222) ● US $255.00

*Novel Applications of Virtual Communities in Healthcare Settings*
Christo El Morr (York University, Canada)
Medical Information Science Reference ● ©2018 ● 247pp ● H/C (ISBN: 9781522529583) ● US $235.00

*Handbook of Research on Data Science for Effective Healthcare Practice and Administration*
Elham Akhond Zadeh Noughabi (University of Calgary, Canada) Bijan Raahemi (University of Ottawa, Canada) Amir Albadvi (Tarbiat Modares University, Iran) and Behrouz H. Far (University of Calgary, Canada)
Medical Information Science Reference ● ©2017 ● 545pp ● H/C (ISBN: 9781522525158) ● US $255.00

*Patent Law and Intellectual Property in the Medical Field*
Rashmi Aggarwal (Institute of Management Technology Ghaziabad, India) and Rajinder Kaur (Panjab University, India)
Medical Information Science Reference ● ©2017 ● 257pp ● H/C (ISBN: 9781522524144) ● US $200.00

*Design, Development, and Integration of Reliable Electronic Healthcare Platforms*
Anastasius Moumtzoglou (P&A Kyriakou Children's Hospital, Greece)
Medical Information Science Reference ● ©2017 ● 357pp ● H/C (ISBN: 9781522517245) ● US $205.00

*For an entire list of titles in this series, please visit:*
*https://www.igi-global.com/book-series/advances-healthcare-information-systems-administration/37156*

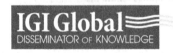

701 East Chocolate Avenue, Hershey, PA 17033, USA
Tel: 717-533-8845 x100 ● Fax: 717-533-8661
E-Mail: cust@igi-global.com ● www.igi-global.com

# Editorial Advisory Board

# Table of Contents

# Detailed Table of Contents

## Chapter 1
IoT in the Field of Healthcare ........................................................... 1
   *K. Govinda, VIT University, India*

The chapter at first focuses on IoT being used in healthcare in general and then it moves to Parkinson's disease, specifically, and how people with it can be benefitted by IoT.

## Chapter 2
Smart Healthcare ................................................................................ 21
   *R. Rajkumar, VIT University, India*

Internet of things is a revolutionary domain, when we use it for the wellness of people in a smart way. As of now, the cost to implement IoT-enabled services is very high. So, this chapter introduces a cost effective and a reliable system to monitor patients at home and in hospitals with the help of IoT. The monitored details of a person can be drawn at any time with the help of an android app, which can produce output at real-time. The processed data are stored in the UBIDOTS cloud server, and the patients' needs can be met in time as well lives saved during critical cases with the help of the system proposed in this chapter.

Cloud computing is an emerging technology that is expected to support internet-scale critical applications, which could be essential to the healthcare sector. Its scalability, resilience, adaptability, connectivity, cost reduction, and high-performance features have high potential to lift the efficiency and quality of healthcare. With the widespread application of healthcare information and communication technology, constructing a stable and sustainable data sharing circumstance has attracted rapidly growing attention in both academic research area and the healthcare industry. Cloud computing is one of long dreamed visions of healthcare cloud (HC), which matches the need of healthcare workers, information sharing directly to various health providers over the internet, regardless of their location and the amount of data. This chapter proposes a cloud model for health information sharing and integration in HC and looks into the arising challenges in healthcare.

Mobile devices are continuously improving, adding integrated sensors, which are of value to the healthcare industry. Sensor-enabled mobile phones collect data from patients, which is useful for doctors in providing immediate care and treatment. As smartphones become ubiquitous, their use as health monitors should become commonplace. This chapter surveys mobile computing devices and sensors in healthcare applications.

Surveillance is defined as providing security in critical situations or monitoring certain places where safety and security are important. Surveillance takes the lead in healthcare departments or sections. Surveillance is also helpful in diagnosing the errors that occur in the automated systems and happening of adverse events in patient care. The main objective of patient surveillance is to observe the changes that occur in any patient's health to provide appropriate medication through automation process. Initially, the comparison is made between surveillance and monitoring.

Later the chapter discusses the wireless technologies and mobile applications used for patient surveillance. Using mobile healthcare systems surveillance data that includes not only patient's clinical information but also analyses clinical scenario periodically, the clinical information gathered is disseminated among various teams of specialists for decision making. The advancement in wireless devices not only monitors the patient's conditions but also provides required information or data. This is possible only when sensed data is communicated at an appropriate time to avoid unexpected events in critical care units. This wireless technology helps the nursing staff in improving the surveillance and guaranteeing patient's safety. This chapter explores mobile patient surveillance.

FHIR standard is designed to enable interoperability and integration with the newest and adopted technologies by the industry. This chapter presents a number of blueprints for the design and development of FHIR servers that enable the integration between HIT systems with m-health applications via FHIR. Each blueprint is based on the location that FHIR servers can be placed with respect to the components of the m-health application (UI, API, server) or a HIT system in order to define and design the necessary infrastructure to facilitate the exchange of information via FHIR. To demonstrate the feasibility of the work, this chapter utilizes the Connecticut concussion tracker (CT2) m-health application as a proof-of-concept prototype that fully illustrates the blueprints of the design and development steps that are involved. The blueprints can be applied to any m-health application and are informative and instructional for medical stakeholders, researchers, and developers.

Nowadays, a person's medical information is just as important as their financial records as they may include not only names and addresses but also various sensitive data such as their employee details, bank account/credit card information, insurance details, etc. However, this fact is often overlooked when designing a file storage system for storing healthcare data. Storage systems are increasingly subject to attacks, so the security system is quickly becoming a mandatory feature of the data storage systems. For the purpose of security, we are dependent on various methods such as cryptographic techniques, two-step verification, and even biometric scanners. This chapter provides a mechanism to create a secure file storage system that provides two-layer security. The first layer is in the form of a password, through which the file is encrypted at the time of storage, and second is the locations at which the user wants the files to be accessed. Thus, this system would allow a user to access a file only at the locations specified by him/her. Therefore, the objective is to create a system that provides secure file storage based on geo-location information.

The most recent couple of decades have seen a sharp rise in the number of elderly individuals. Furthermore, enquiry into this tells us that around 89% of the matured individuals are probably going to live autonomously. As the need be, giving a respectable personal satisfaction for matured individuals has turned into a genuine social test. Doctors need to have clear idea as to the health of these individuals, so they can use proper methodologies to cure them. Hence, IoT develops the idea of the internet and makes it more unavoidable. IoT permits consistent collaborations among various sorts of gadgets, for example, therapeutic sensors, observing cameras, home machines, and so on. This chapter proposes clinical data analysis using the internet of things.

Recent technological advances in wireless communications and wireless sensor networks have enabled the design of intelligent, tiny, low-cost, and lightweight medical sensor nodes that can be placed on the human body strategically. The focus of this chapter is to implement the health monitoring system continuously without hospitalization using wearable sensors and create a wireless body area network (WBAN). Wearable sensors monitor the parameters of the human body like temperature, pressure, and heart beat by using sensors and providing real-time feedback to the user and medical staff and WBANs promise to revolutionize health monitoring. In this chapter, medical sensors are used to collect physiological data from patients and transmit it to the system which has details of an individual stored using Bluetooth/Wi-Fi with the help of Arduino and to medical server using Wi-Fi/3G communications.

Internet of things is where all the things are connected to the internet and communicate with each other. There are many applications of the IoT in various fields such as healthcare, agriculture, industries, and logistics, and even for empowering people with disabilities. There are many previous work for the blind people using IoT in finding the obstacles many navigation applications have been developed. In this chapter, a system is proposed to assist blind people in reading books. This method is based on capturing the text book pages as an image and processing them into text with speech as an output.

# Preface

The use of mobile devices by healthcare professionals (HCPs) has transformed many aspects of clinical practice. Mobile devices have become commonplace in healthcare settings, leading to rapid growth in the development of medical software applications (apps) for these platforms. Numerous apps are now available to assist HCPs with many important tasks, such as: information and time management; health record maintenance and access; communications and consulting; reference and information gathering; patient management and monitoring; clinical decision-making; and medical education and training. Mobile devices and apps provide many benefits for HCPs, perhaps most significantly increased access to point-of-care tools, which has been shown to support better clinical decision-making and improved patient outcomes. However, some HCPs remain reluctant to adopt their use. Despite the benefits they offer, better standards and validation practices regarding mobile medical apps need to be established to ensure the proper use and integration of these increasingly sophisticated tools into medical practice. These measures will raise the barrier for entry into the medical app market, increasing the quality and safety of the apps currently available for use by HCPs.

This Healthcare Mobile Applications aims to be an essential reference source, helpful in building on the available resource in the field of Healthcare and in developing countries while providing for further research opportunities in this Healthcare field. It is hoped that this text will provide the resources necessary for Healthcare professionals, Patients, Hospital Administrators to adopt and implement Mobile Apps for healthcare in developing nations across the globe.

# TARGET AUDIENCE

Healthcare Professionals, Academicians, Researchers, Hospital administrators, Research-level students, Doctors, Technology developers, Healthcare Professionals will find this text useful in furthering their research exposure to pertinent topics in electronic government and assisting in furthering their own research efforts in this field.

Chapter 1 focuses on IoT being used in Healthcare in general and then it moves to the Parkinson's disease and how people who woe from it can be benefitted with the help of IoT. Chapter 2 we are introducing a cost effective and a reliable system to monitor the patients at home and in hospitals with the help of IoT. The monitored details of a person can be drawn at any time with the help of an android app which can produce output at real-time. The processed data arc stored in the ubidots cloud server and the patient needs can be met in time as well as saves life. Chapter 3 proposes cloud model for health information sharing and integration in HC and look into the arising challenges in healthcare.

In Chapter 4 we discuss the interaction between users, computer and machine used in day to day activities. The mobile which is very useful for voice communication and messaging services, taking pictures and playing videos etc. These services will be utilized towards development of mobile healthcare activities. Chapter 5 focuses on patient safety in critical and acute units of hospitals. Later the chapter discusses the roles of nurse interventions, the existing strategies and identifying risks in advance. Surveillance data include not only patient's clinical information but also analyses clinical scenario periodically. To make the patient monitoring system function successfully, wireless technology is needed.

Chapter 6 presents a number of blueprints for the design and development of FHIR servers that enable the integration between HIT systems with mHealth applications via FHIR. Each blueprint is based on the location that FHIR servers can be placed with respect to the components of the mHealth application (UI, API, and Server) or a HIT system in order to define and design the necessary infrastructure to facilitate the exchange of information via FHIR.

Chapter 7 provides two layered security. The first layer is in the form of a password using which the file is encrypted at the time of storage and second is the locations at which the user wants the files to be accessed. This system would allow a user to access a file only at the locations specified by the user. The objective is to create a system that provides secure file storage based on geolocation information. Chapter 8 focuses on clinical data analysis using internet of things. IoT permits consistent collaborations among various sorts of gadgets, for example, therapeutic sensor, observing cameras, home machines so on. Chapter 9's focus is to implement the health monitoring system continuously without hospitalization using wearable sensors and create a wireless body area network (WBAN). Wearable sensors monitor the parameters of the human body like temperature, pressure, heart beat by using sensors and providing real-time feedback to the user and medical staff and WBANs promise to revolutionize health monitoring. In Chapter 10, a system is proposed for the blind people in assisting them in reading the books. This method is based on capturing the text book pages as an image and processing them in to text with a speech as an output.

# Acknowledgment

I would like to express my gratitude to the many people helped me in writing this book. I would like to thank all those who provided support and offered comments, allowed and assisted me in editing, proofreading and design.

I would like to thank our Honourable Chancellor Dr. G. Viswanathan VIT University for enabling me to publish this book. Above all I want to thank my wife, Dr. P. K. Lincy, my daughters R. R. Dhisha, R. R. Dia and of my family, who supported and encouraged me in spite of all the time it took me away from them. It was a long and difficult journey for them.

I would like to thank all my authors and reviewers who contributed for helping me in the process of selection and editing. Last and not least: I beg forgiveness of all those who have been with me over the course of the years and whose names I have failed to mention."

I am grateful to all of those with whom I have had the pleasure to work with during this and other related projects. I would especially like to thank my Holy Cross Matriculation school friends and teachers. As my teacher and mentor, they have taught me more than I could ever give them credit for here.

*R. Rajkumar*
*VIT University, India*

# Introduction

The purpose of this book is to help educate the public on how Healthcare Applications can be done with mobile, to show the components of a system, and to eliminate the idea that the process is complex. The author has had multiple requests for healthcare information, which demonstrated a need of mobile in healthcare to get the patients information purposes. Several state manuals and international books exist for the subject, but no one book/document is as comprehensive with mobile, healthcare, simulations, details, and references.

## AUDIENCE

The audience for this book ranges from a beginner looking to collect information for healthcare professionals like doctors, nurses, health inspectors or a future mobile APP project to a more knowledgeable system. An excellent reference and resource section is provided for a reader to expand the knowledge provided in the book to allow the advance Mobile APP & Cloud system to gain even additional information.

## MESSAGE(S)

The message of the book is that it is time to wake up and realize we have a sensors mobile which are most widely used by everyone Mobile Sensors that is slowly being depleted and unless we start to take care of it, we will experience lack of new technologies like other part of the world are currently experiencing. A second underlying message is that designers specifically work on healthcare projects which incorporate passive techniques.

# Chapter 1
# IoT in the Field of Healthcare

**K. Govinda**
*VIT University, India*

## ABSTRACT

*The chapter at first focuses on IoT being used in healthcare in general and then it moves to Parkinson's disease, specifically, and how people with it can be benefitted by IoT.*

## INTRODUCTION

Technology, over the years has always brought about a revolutionary change in the history of mankind. Be it good or bad, it has always influenced us in a large way and has shaped the modern 21st century world. Though it has led to war and destruction, it has also helped keep world peace and unity. Over the years, mankind has seen many interesting and breathtaking discoveries which have revolutionized the different aspects of everyday life. The Internet of Things is one such topic which has evolved or rather come across a long way since its discovery in the 90's. It has pioneered the way for headway and development. It has connected various people across the globe and has led to path breaking discoveries and countless inventions which aims to provide a better future for all of us. It has conquered many fields including science, medicine. Smart objects inspired by IoT are found in each and every walks of life such as Smart Homes, Smart Parking System, Smart Agriculture etc. The IoT is an ideal technology which has played a key role in communication. We have seen that through the years how internet became the base for various programs. In this world of IoT, each object which has been connected, be

DOI: 10.4018/978-1-5225-5036-5.ch001

it a phone or a room etc is considered to be smart. It has been programmed in such a way that it can be used to its utmost capabilities with the help of existing technologies such as RFID etc.

Smart Healthcare is very important in various health related applications through various sensors in patients and their medicines for seeing upon them. The IoT is used by clinical care to take care of the physiological and neurological conditions of the unhealthy through sensors by amassing their existing status and then passing this information to the required centers so that the doctors can check upon these affected people and take necessary steps in order to prevent deterioration of the patient's condition. For example, if the blood pressure of a heart patient is varying rapidly, this can easily be detected by certain important sensors which will then process this information and send it to the concerned authorities who can take immediate action to prevent any mishaps and ensure the safety of the person. Various patients in hospitals require proper attention and they can be checked upon using IoT inspired monitoring. This method deploys sensors to accumulator important physiological information and uses gateways to get the job done. When you go to your medical exam, The doctor not only has general clinical / laboratory testing was based on static dimensions of your biological and metabolic, but also abundant better data from sensors. Using presented data, and assisted by verdict support schemes also will be having admittance to a large amount of observational data for other people have, your neurologist can make a much superior prognosis of the health and advise on treatment. Such a troublesome expertise with a transformational influence on could have worldwide fitness schemes and a radical decrease in healthcare costs and recover the haste and precision of analysis. In day to day life where everyone is busy, where we don't have much span to check and to keep a watch on everything. How do we intend to keep our health good? Sensors offer us with correct and proper output and it's a much better selection than ancient medical instruments like thermometers like they may have optical phenomenon errors. For endlessly sending message from person's location to medical informative GSM electronic equipment is used. Now days, heart diseases are exceeds up to dangerous level which results in death of such a large amount of individuals. Observance of patient anytime is tough or doctors also are unable to observe explicit patient for total operating hours. In several important conditions like patient is found remote from hospital or conjointly just in case of old patient who suffering with heart condition and physical disorders, continuous observance of patient isn't potential (Ufoaroh, Oranugo, & Uchechukwu, 2015).

These days, the health care sensors are assuming an essential part in our everyday life. Health care checking frameworks is one of the real upgrades in view of its advanced innovation. So we are essentially interfacing the temperature sensor and heart rate sensor so that at the same time we can observe the state of person who have been suffering and subsequently discounting the utilization of the thermometer and different devices to check the present state of the person who have been suffering.

A heart rate sensor is an individual measuring device for individuals and it enables the subject to check his/her present heart rate for further examination. Prior Systems were included a container that contains terminal leads which are connected to the chest. Grown-ups show at least a bit of kindness rate roughly around 72 beats for every moment (bpm) and for children it's around 120bpm. A few more seasoned kids have heart rates around 90 bpm. The heart rate rises step by step amid activities and backs off to rest an incentive after exercise (Jubadi, & Sahak, 2009). In the event that the rate at which the beat comes back with the ordinary estimation of heart rate, then it implies that the specific individual is fit. Individuals with heart rates lower than the typical are generally confronting a condition known as bradycardia, while the general population with higher face a condition which is known as tachycardia. Heart rate is basically figured by keeping the fingertip to the LDR sensor and afterward assessing and including the beats for the most part a 30 seconds of a specific time period (Jadhav, Devkatte, & Dhumal, 2015; Kale, A. V., Gawade, Jadhav, & Patil, 2015). The specific domain name for this application would be: It would be used to detect heart rate and body temperature. It would be used to detect fever and help us to state how much stressed up we are and how much exercise we need.

In a broader context it would be a part of "MEDICAL SCIENECE". The main Moto is to develop a Heart Rate and Temperature Monitoring System which could help those people who have been suffering from heart rate and physical disorder. This paper deals with solving above problems. Module consist of wireless sensor which measures the heart rate and body temperature and sends the value of heartbeat and temperature to the android phone with the help of Bluetooth module. If there is any abnormalities then SMS will be send through GSM module to the medical advisory for the precautions so that patient can be prevented from serious health problem or serious situation before reaching to the hospital. For display the measured values of heart beat and body temperature, LCD is used. From android phone, it will be also sent to the cloud database.

The evolution of technology has been inching towards a more integrated, connected environment and society. Each new invention, discovery or development is leading to an overall improvement in the quality of life for each human being. There is an increase in the life expectancy of each person and consequently, the progressive ageing of the human race. There are several side effects and drawbacks of this whole process as well. The swift upsurge in the number of people affected by chronic diseases has been the topic of several conversations. Additionally, the increase in life expectancy also means there is an upsurge in the number of elderlies who require palliative care and attention from caregivers or doctors. As more and more people have begun to live alone, not only is regular monitoring and nursing difficult for each person, personal support and care is progressively challenging to provide one to one upkeep for all. In the case of any emergency, the first responders can only respond only after the victim raises an alarm that he is in distress. This is not a very proactive approach for a technology driven world. To ensure a decent quality of life, we must ensure remote access of such health data and vital signs of a person to adopt an active tactic in observing and maintaining the personal health of anybody. By integrating IoT-enabled devices in medical equipment, healthcare professionals are able to monitor their patients very effectively. They can also and the data collected from these devices to determine which patients require the most active attention. In different words, by making the most of this network of devices, healthcare specialists may use data to create a system of pre-emptive management – as is often said by a lot of people, the prevention is better than the cure.

IoT based remote monitoring tools have hence become central to a shift in paradigm in the healthcare industry to adapt to these new upcoming needs of people. The quantification of human health conditions can be done discretely by now inexpensive, wearable sensors that can measure various vital signs of any human being and transmit over short or long range to the appropriate medical personnel who can interpret this data and immediately respond. In many cases, systems are also designed to perform actuation on the basis of recorded signs. These new, cheap, wearable sensors have the potential to establish the Smart-health systems for various classes and categories of patients like those suffering from chronic fatal and non-fatal diseases, the elderly and even more so for people who want to monitor their health on a regular basis. The sensors are attached to various parts of the body of a person to monitor vitals such as heartbeat, blood glucose levels, body temperature, blood pressure, etc. and transmit the data for statistical analysis so as to deduce behavioral patterns of a person and enable professional to advice and guide them on how to improve health practices. Besides, such systems can also set off alarms and prompt for remote action and provide adequate help at the right time to all those who need it in times of emergency. This shall go a long way in improving life expectancy and is also a cost-effective way of maintaining regular patient records in hospitals and health centers.

The greater part of the budding countries has exceptionally bad healthcare transportation. There are very less doctor's facilities in contrast with blasting population. That couple of doctor's facilities is insufficiently prepared and not many specialists are available for the essential diagnostic equipment used for finding of life frightening diseases is missing. On the off chance that if we can construct cheaper convenient health sensing device, including a few sensors, fit for measuring the key traits of a human body, and can speak with the hospital database, we could furnish with excellent medicinal counsel.

The health check is given after the authority specialists from the gathering of specific specialists there throughout the world assess those health constraints on clinic database. It acts as private cloud. Besides, if healthcare sensing gadget is made to speak among convenient PC like a tab or cell phone which have default capacity of speaking with the clinic database, in that case, the entire framework will be considerably extra financially suitable. This is on the grounds that these days a great many people have entry to convenient communication devices and these gadgets have turned out to be very cost effective. The framework can likewise has prepared IoT empowered and M2M friendly.

This paper displays the usage of healthcare monitoring system. In this manner, we can possibly profit a vast population. Every sensor ought to timely compute the information taking after the approved sampling time of the constraint, and information ought to be sending to the information processor with no overlap used for healthcare monitoring system to become dependable. Every sensor has differing prerequisites regarding information length and sampling speed the sensor information gathered without overlap by information processor we can replace notepad at patient bed with smart device by utilizing NFC technology and patient's information can be extricated from smart gadget consequently by utilizing NFC.

IoT is the next era of human life (Free Scale and Emerging Technologies, ARM, 2016), IoT is no more a hype it has started to become a reality (Evans, 2011; Zanella, Bui, Castellani, Vangelista, & Zorzi, 2014), IoT has changed the human thinking in all the aspects of life (ITU-T Technology Watch Report, 2013), IoT is converting normal cities to smart cities (Borodin, Zavyalova,

Zaharov, & Yamushev, 2015; La, Kim, & Kim, 2015), IoT uses a lot of RFID tags, sensors and cloud servers for its functioning.

In (Catarinucci, De Donno, Mainetti, Palano, Patrono, Stefanizzi, & Tarricone, 2015) *ecg* and heart rate are monitored with the help of a app where the data's are stored in local storage and in cloud memory and can keep an eye on the patients' health progress. In (Rahmani, Thanigaivelan, Gia, Granados, Negash, Liljeberg, & Tenhunen, 2015) we are monitoring diseases like hypertension, diabetes and *ecg* they are integrated in a sensor kit. The outcome values can be monitored on desktop. The introduction of a smart gateway where the data from the sensors are stored in the cloud *db* and user *db*. All the data's are received from the sensors through wireless medium (Seales, Do, Belyi, & Kumar, 2015). Data's are stored in the cloud server through internet web clients can use smart phones and laptops to see the data of the accelerometer and *ecg* are made in this paper (Gope & Hwang, 2016) but a power efficient one. With the help of *phinet*as the cloud service we integrate all the actions performed values from the sensors like accelerometer, temperature,*ecg* and air flow sensor can be visualizes by healthcare professionals (Chiuchisan, Chiuchisan, & Dimian, 2015). BSN body sensor network where we monitor details of sensor like *eeg*, *emg*, Blood Pressure, Motion Detection, *ecg* and temperature with the help of internet to the *bsn* care server where the local physicians and emergency team will take care of them (Serdaroglu, Uslu, & Baydere, 2015). In (Gupta, Patchava, & Menezes, 2015) we monitor the blood pressure, pulse and oxygen, electrocardiogram, patient position and body temperature with the help of the microcontroller to the clients like doctor, family, friends and emergency team with the help of internet and also as implementation of mobile app. Activity recognition has been implemented for the patients to monitor whether the elderly persons are taking pills or the medications at the right time prescribed by the physicians with the help of *rfid* tag and reader. If the person is inactive during the prescribed time an alert will be sent to the admin. Electrocardiogram is used to sense the health of the patient and monitor it updates the values at regular intervals to the website. Forwarding the values as a message to the doctor if any abnormal value is found and also turning on the buzzer. This new technology with advantages brings in a lot of disadvantages along with it.In this paper we discuss the advantages and disadvantages involved by getting IoT into our day to day life and conclude if IoT is a boon or curse to healthcare.

## BACKGROUND

Over the years, several papers have focused on the healthcare benefits in general. They have mentioned various cases about how IoT has played about a major role in the betterment of the sick, diseased and the unhealthy.

One of the papers written in the IEEE Conference on Overhaul Computing spoke about Health Nursing and Administration using the Internet of Things. The writers enlightened us as to how Networked sensors make it possible to gather large amount of data which tells us about the psychological and corporeal health. Apprehended on an extensive period basis, combined, and successfully administered, such data could transmit about a sole and delightful alteration in the vigor care domain. In specific, the handiness of figures at impossible balances and chronological length attached with a first-hand cohort of bright procedures can: (a) ease an development in the recurrence of therapeutic stadium, from the contemporary pole facto diagnose-and treat sensitive example, to an astounding practice for analysis of these various ailments, coupled with discouragement, cure, and the slow development of fitness instead of syndrome; (b) empower personalizing of conduct and administration options beleaguered chiefly to the particular conditions and wanting of the separate; and (c) help substantiate the fee of health care while concurrently refining aftermaths. In this paper, the icing on the cake will be the chances and encounters with IoT in seeing this revelation of the forthcoming health care regions.

The IoT plays a important role in a comprehensive range of healthcare solicitations, from managing chronic diseases to avert diseases. Here are some examples of how its role is already being seen:

## Clinical

Hospitalized people whose biological status necessitates close care can be frequently monitored using IoT driven, noninvasive observing. This type of answer employs antennae to collect ample physiological statistics and uses posterns and the cloud to scrutinize and store information to caregivers for additional analysis and evaluation. It substitutes the procedure of consuming a health professional come by at steady intermissions to check the patient's vigorous signs, instead if a continuous automated flow of evidence. In this way, it instantaneously advances the superiority of care through thoughtfulness and depresses the cost of maintenance by eradicating the need for a caregiver to energetically engage in info assembly and anaysis.

## Remote Checking

There are folks all over the realm whose health may agonize because they don't have complete access to current health observing. But small, authoritative wireless solutions connected over the IoT are now building it possible for watching to come to these patients instead of vice versa. These resolutions can be castoff to steadily imprisonment patient data. A variation of sensors and apply composite algorithms in order to examine the data. The progress achieved in this field has been mind-boggling and has helped ease the pain endured due to lack of proper healthcare facilities.

Figure 1 shows us one of the current trends used in the field of healthcare with the help of the various components of IoT such as sensors (temperature, humidity, vibration etc).

- **Parkinson's Disease:** Parkinson's disease (PD) is a continuing and broadminded program ailment, meaning that indicators endure and deteriorate over period. Nearly around two million individuals in the country of India are bodily with Parkinson's disease. The origin is strange, and even though nearby is presently no remedy, there might be management options for example prescription and surgery to cope its indications. Parkinson's begins with the diminishing of vivacious nerve cells in the cerebrum, called neurons. Parkinson's to a great extent influences these particular nerve cells in a zone of the mind named the substantianigra. As PD upgrades, the condition of the person deteriorates over time which leads to a person not able to control his movements.

*Figure 1.*

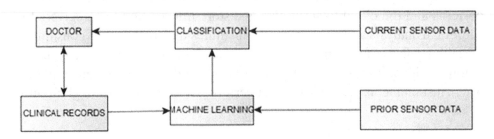

Effects of Parkinson's include:

1. Quiver of the hands and feet,
2. Not able to perform day to day activities.

The choice of PD be represented by upon the being of at least one of the four most mutual engine side effects of the sickness. In including, there are other minor and teetotaler proposals that touch numerous people and are logically familiar by clinicians as crucial to giving Parkinson's.

By definition, Parkinson's is a dynamic sickness. Albeit a few people with Parkinson's just have markers on one side of the figure for innumerable years, in the long run the signs start on the extra side. Signs on the additional side of the frame regularly don't change over as unembellished as signs on the early transversely.

The aim of this paper, is on the heartbeat rate monitoring and to alert the person and it is also able to observe the heart rate abnormality of a person. The system concludes and then sends an alert text to the mobile phone. It is compact and cost effective. It is very efficient system thus easy to handle and hence provides greater flexibility and serves as an improvement over other customary monitoring and alert systems. Biomedical engineering (BME) it has two angles: the design and the problem resolving techniques of engineering combined with medical sciences to enhance patient's wellbeing and the quality of life of individuals. The primary and a very common reason to ultimate death in the world are the cardiovascular diseases. The only feasible tool for the diagnosis is the heart beat readings that could aid early detection of cardiac events. We can measure one's heart rate through fingertip by this method.

The essential wireless technologies that as of now are used for social insurance frameworks are RFID, Bluetooth, ZigBee and remote sensor network which gives creative medium for information transmission in the field of medicine. WBAN ordinarily utilizes Zigbee. The smart sensors dealt with by patients transmit fundamental signs and flags to individual server consecutively; the information is transmitted from individual server to servers of the healthcare framework, similar to weather forecast, medical database or crisis server over Internet. Calculations might be executed on the healthcare framework servers to give moment and patient-particular proposals.

In the paper, the existing research is evaluated on wireless body area network in Healthcare framework. By utilizing wban health related medicinal services, framework will build up their performa and will be helpful for decreasing death rate. This give Quality of Service, low power utilization, consistent wellbeing observing and portability. In proposed framework they are processing the heart rate and body temperature variables by utilizing key elements of wireless body area network. In which data are taken from sensors which are sent on to android cell phone and subsequent to figuring down those data, heart assault can be normal. With the goal that versatility is achieved, and telemedicine framework is additionally implemented (Mazidi, McKinlay, & Causey, 2008).

In this paper, Patient Monitoring System using wireless technology strengthens the capabilities of doctors and medical authorities to track patient's vital conditions and determine their health condition. Persistent screen are the most essential symptomatic gadgets in basic care units of healing facilities that gives ceaseless show and translation of the patient's crucial parameters. Patient monitoring system measures physiological condition either continuously or at regular interval. The patient's monitoring requirements includes periodic detection of routine vital parameters and transmission of alerting signals when vital parameter indicates any type of threats or danger. PMS has resulted in stronger bedside patient monitors which are adequate of complex bio-signal processing.

In this paper, 12V and 5V power supply given to GSM modem and different gadgets individually. At the point when framework will begin, all devices are initialized. At that point heart rate sensor and temperature sensor measures heart rate and body temperature individually and both yields are given to the PIC controller. By means of GSM modem with the assistance of AT-Commands this data sends to medical authority. In the middle of PIC controller and GSM level converter is utilized to change over TTL to CMOS level and the other way around. For level changing over reason, we utilized MAX232 IC. In this module, we are given limit level for heart rate and body temperature. When heart rate and body gets temperature exceeded abnormally then the buzzer will turns ON (AmolGosavi, Dnyaneshwar Kandekar, Ghadge, Behere, & Patil) Pic controller gets easy program updates and it is small in size. Machinery and control system are the major use of PICI6F877A (Pounraj, Winston, Christabel, & Ramaraj, 2016).

When we placed a finger on heart rate sensor, it gives its output. The led sensor will blink up on each heartbeat. The sensor output is directly associated to PIC controller to calculate the heart beat rate. It is based on the phenomenon of blood flowing through fingertip at each pulse. LED is use in to detect the blood flowing through the vessels (Sundaram, 2013).

Advancement in the field of Micro Electro Mechanical Systems (MEMS) has led to a lot of imminent progression in the study of WSNs. There is a lot of existing research in the field of wireless sensors networks used in various applications. They have several uses in many different industries. Some of them include military applications, security and health. in the military, they have been used for various specific purposes such as battlefield surveillance and battle damage assessment. Existing research in collection of physiological data from wireless sensors nodes to transmit to doctors or medical personnel has been exhaustive. Several applications have been designed for various purposes such as patient tracking, drug administration and tele monitoring of patient's data over the web. WSNs have been very convenient in usage for ambient assisted living applications as well. WSNs can also been used to check chemical levels and water purity levels in pollution check systems. They aid in detecting amount of pollutants and chemicals in water or air. They can also be used to check the amount of nutrients in the soil which is extremely useful and beneficial in agricultural applications as well. Other applications also include home automation and home security systems. Wireless sensor nodes have been deployed in a wide variety of applications. They have been widely researched. One the major advantages of wireless sensors are their low power consumption compared to other modes of communication. According to several researchers, these systems are also largely fault tolerant. They also solve the issue of wiring and restricting the mobility of the systems they are attached.

The following aspect would clarify about the proposed smart health monitoring and alert system. There are such a variety of places where this system is utilized. This is for the most part utilized as a part of the places where medical centre are far away.

This paper describes the health monitoring system for PV array of 2×2 . This method is used for finding the health position of patient in 30 mins. from 6.00 am to 6.00 pm. This method is used for improvement of extraction of energy, it detects the fault accurately and it is extendable for any kind of arrays. It can implement the reconfigured control switch for the increase of power generation of the faulty conditions of this system (Spencer Jr, Ruiz-Sandoval, & Kurata, 2004).

This paper describes the monitoring of ECG, heart rate, SpO2, pulse rate and temperature by using a patient's health monitoring system. The values are uploaded in a web server by storing them in a database In future; it can be uploaded in a database automatically. The doctor who is sitting abroad can also get the full report of patient's medical history so that they can see and advice the patient that what they can do for the treatment of the disease (Navya, & Murthy, 2013).

This paper gave a prologue to smart sensing technology, recognizing various occasions, and a portion of the related difficulties. Smart sensors which are on the Mote worldview will give the capacity to improvement of the up and coming era of structural health monitoring frameworks and opens new prospects for innovative work. Multi-specialist system innovation presents a computational structure for new calculations execution (Setyowati, Muninggar, & NA, 2017).

The paper describes a Wireless Sensor Network (WSN) used for observing patient's physiological circumstances continually utilizing Zigbee. In this paper, the physiological values, for example, body temperature, heart rate, body effect and saline level are observed. Low-control arranged intensifiers were utilized to limit battery utilization. The design of the IR sensors could be upgraded to diminishing its acceptance to buzz, to a point where it could be moved onto the wrist unit. The unit is intended for use by the develop, inside the house, where a caretaker is available yet is not ready to be always in visual contact with the patient (Perera, Liu, & Jayawardena, 2015).

In this paper, the healthcare monitoring is prepared by utilizing remote sensor gadgets and reports all the sensor information to the doctor. Throughout the healthcare monitoring if any patient wellbeing condition is severe, then it sends a crisis notice message to the doctor by utilizing GSM innovation. Utilizing four sensors connected to healthcare monitoring, for example, beat sensor, Accelerometer, breathing sensor and blood Pressure sensor which is controlled by microcontroller and get information from sensors. The work left will be intended to utilize Zigbee to send information from sensor gadgets to PC and they will utilize GSM innovation to send crisis notice messages to the doctor's mobile (Arpan Pal, Innovation Lab, 2016).

## Proposed Approach

For many persons breathing with Parkinson's disease, the performance of mastication and believing can be a test. One way to contract with this is to mixture foods up to minimalist the essential to portion. But what if it's problematic just bringing the serve to one's mouth without dropping its fillings? In order to target this, I have thought of a few devices that not only help to counter Parkinson's disease but also make the lives of those affected much easier with the help of this.

## Smart Pen/Spoon

Smart Pen is the first tremor stopping pen that syndicates software and hardware to make a clever resolution to the extensively knowledgeable problematic of script tremors. It uses dynamic steadying to counterbalance tremors much more meritoriously than key snow on the market. Inside, a gimbals instrument

*Figure 2. IMU: An inertial measurement unit (IMU) is an electrical device that processes and reports a body's exact force, angular rate by means of able no. of accelerometers*

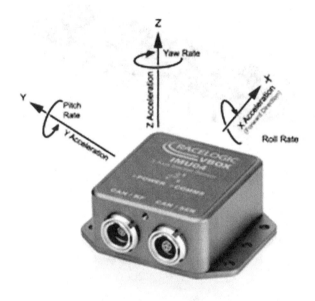

*Figure 3. Tilt and Accelerometer Sensors: Orientation sensing*

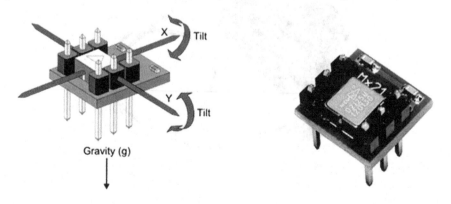

and a equipoise regulator procedure work in tandem to mollify the pen. Make the calligraphy tremor-free. The pen is also malleable. By substituting the insert with any inscription utensil, all kinds of doings can advantage from the pen's single soothing skills.

A servomotor is a rotary actuator that countenances for detailed control of angular or linear position, velocity and acceleration.

*Figure 4. 8 Bit AVR Microcontroller*

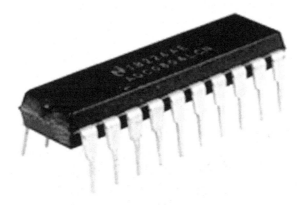

*Figure 5. Servo Motor*

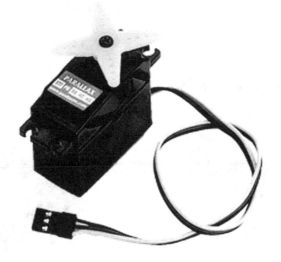

## Working

The person's tremors are checked upon by the system which goes as an acceleration data which is taken from the IMU and then passes through (AVR) which executes guesstimate on the data assimilated from the acceleration sensor. In order to make sure that the system will go in an opposite directional electromagnetic (a servo) drive is premeditated to function with an embedded micro-controller based application. Every time there is a change in acceleration data the servo is actuated in a direction opposite to the recorded value from the person's hand tremor. This device uses six-point based sensor data calibration (Ufoaroh, Oranugo, & Uchechukwu, 2015).

## Smart Devices to Improve Voice

Apps and devices can give individuals more control over the choice of therapy plans. The idea is to create an app that changes the frequency of the voice of the person suffering from Parkinson's disease. It is highly suitable for improving loudness or for normalizing speech rate.

## Walking Device

(Smart) Falls are an intermittent and perilous inconvenience of Parkinson's infection. Understanding reviews show that the rate of PWPs who learning falls can keep running as high as 68 percent. Parkinson's patients are at an expanded danger of dropping due to the signs of Parkinson's sickness - strong solidness, solidifying, rearranging stride, adjust debilitation or stooped stance - and in uncommon cases thus of the reactions of anti-parking son meds. Indeed, even a minor fall can starting point wounds and sprains. More mindful falls can reason genuine wounds, for example, destroyed bones or electronic stun. In totaling, the fear of decreasing can likewise touch PWP enthusiastic, which unwillingness to authorization the family unit. In this way, Fall Deterrence is a huge guideline for giving Parkinson's sickness, extraordinarily exposed to the harsh elements months, when even garages and walkways require additional safety measures. Here we plot a portion of the proposals would come. In order to counter this, a smart walking device can be formed which senses the movement of the person and prevents him from falling by tilting in a particular direction.

## Smart Room

Equipping the room to an ambient temperature and ensuring that the patient is taken care of properly.

Figure 6 provides the working of the Smart Spoon.

## CONCLUSION

In this chapter, we have seen how the evolution of healthcare under the influence of IoT has helped the greater humanity at large and what the current

*Figure 6.*

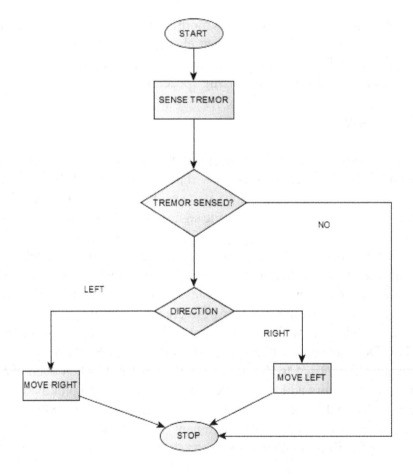

trends are. It particularly focuses on the Parkinson's disease and how it can be tackled if not cured with the help of the Internet of Things.

## Feature Enhancement

Mobile cloud computing (mcc) is able to save energy, improve application and experience of the users. All frameworks mentioned above have their own benefits and issues but still not up to level to address all issues related to security, energy and user experience. Security issues are key problem in mcc, they need to be focused more compare to other issues.

## REFERENCES

Benharref, A., & Serhani, M. A. (2014). Novel cloud and SOA-based framework for E-Health monitoring using wireless biosensors. *IEEE Journal of Biomedical and Health Informatics*, *18*(1), 46–55. doi:10.1109/JBHI.2013.2262659 PMID:24403403

Borodin, A., Zavyalova, Y., Zaharov, A., & Yamushev, I. (2015, April). Architectural approach to the multisource health monitoring application design. In *Open Innovations Association (FRUCT), 2015 17th Conference of* (pp. 16-21). IEEE. 10.1109/FRUCT.2015.7117965

Catarinucci, L., De Donno, D., Mainetti, L., Palano, L., Patrono, L., Stefanizzi, M. L., & Tarricone, L. (2015). An IoT-Aware Architecture for Smart Healthcare Systems. *Internet of Things Journal, IEEE*, *2*(6), 515–526. doi:10.1109/JIOT.2015.2417684

Chiuchisan, I., Chiuchisan, I., & Dimian, M. (2015, October). Internet of Things for e-Health: An approach to medical applications. In *Computational Intelligence for Multimedia Understanding (IWCIM), 2015 International Workshop on* (pp. 1-5). IEEE.

Evans, D. (2011). The internet of things: How the next evolution of the internet is changing everything. *CISCO White Paper*, *1*(2011), 1-11.

Gope, P., & Hwang, T. (2016). BSN-Care: A secure IoT-based modern healthcare system using body sensor network. *IEEE Sensors Journal*, *16*(5), 1368–1376. doi:10.1109/JSEN.2015.2502401

Gupta, M. S. D., Patchava, V., & Menezes, V. (2015, October). Healthcare based on IoT using Raspberry Pi. In *Green Computing and Internet of Things (ICGCIoT), 2015 International Conference on* (pp. 796-799). IEEE. 10.1109/ICGCIoT.2015.7380571

ITU-T Technology watch report. (2013). *Smart cities Seoul: A case study.* Author.

Jadhav, P., Devkatte, B., & Dhumal, V. (2015). The health care monitoring using android mobile phone. *IJETT, 2*(1).

Jubadi, W. M., & Sahak, S. F. A. M. (2009, October). Heartbeat monitoring alert via SMS. In *Industrial Electronics & Applications, 2009. ISIEA 2009. IEEE Symposium on* (Vol. 1, pp. 1-5). IEEE. 10.1109/ISIEA.2009.5356491

Kale, A. V., Gawade, S. D., Jadhav, S. Y., & Patil, S. A. (2015). GSM Based Heart Rate and Temperature Monitoring System. *International Journal of Engineering Research & Technology, 4*(4).

Kale, A. V., Gawade, S. D., Jadhav, S. Y., & Patil, S. A. (2015). GSM Based Heart Rate and Temperature Monitoring System. *International Journal of Engineering Research & Technology, 4*(04).

La, H. J., Kim, M. K., & Kim, S. D. (2015, June). A Personal Healthcare System with Inference-as-a-Service. In *Services Computing (SCC), 2015 IEEE International Conference on* (pp. 249-255). IEEE. 10.1109/SCC.2015.42

Mazidi, M. A., McKinlay, R. D., & Causey, D. (2008). *PIC microcontroller and embedded systems: using Assembly and C for PIC18.* Academic Press.

Natarajan, K., Prasath, B., & Kokila, P. (2016). Smart health care system using internet of things. *Journal of Network Communications and Emerging Technologies, 6*(3).

Navya, K., & Murthy, M. B. R. (2013). A zigbee based patient health monitoring system. *Int. Journal of Engineering Research and Applications, 3*(5).

Pal, A. (2016). Internet of things making the hype a reality. Innovation Lab, Tata Consultancy Services.

Perera, C., Liu, C. H., & Jayawardena, S. (2015). The emerging internet of things marketplace from an industrial perspective: A survey. *IEEE Transactions on Emerging Topics in Computing, 3*(4), 585–598. doi:10.1109/TETC.2015.2390034

Pounraj, P., Winston, D. P., Christabel, S. C., & Ramaraj, R. (2016). A Continuous Health Monitoring System for Photovoltaic Array Using Arduino Microcontroller. *Circuits and Systems*, *7*(11), 3494–3503. doi:10.4236/cs.2016.711297

Rahmani, A. M., Thanigaivelan, N. K., Gia, T. N., Granados, J., Negash, B., Liljeberg, P., & Tenhunen, H. (2015, January). Smart e-health gateway: Bringing intelligence to internet-of-things based ubiquitous healthcare systems. In *Consumer Communications and Networking Conference (CCNC), 2015 12th Annual IEEE* (pp. 826-834). IEEE. 10.1109/CCNC.2015.7158084

Seales, C., Do, T., Belyi, E., & Kumar, S. (2015, June). PHINet: A Plug-n-Play Content-centric Testbed Framework for Health-Internet of Things. In *Mobile Services (MS), 2015 IEEE International Conference on* (pp. 368-375). IEEE. 10.1109/MobServ.2015.57

Serdaroglu, K., Uslu, G., & Baydere, S. (2015, October). Medication intake adherence with real time activity recognition on IoT. In *Wireless and Mobile Computing, Networking and Communications (WiMob), 2015 IEEE 11th International Conference on* (pp. 230-237). IEEE. 10.1109/WiMOB.2015.7347966

Setyowati, V., & Muninggar, J. (2017, January). Design of heart rate monitor based on piezoelectric sensor using an Arduino. *Journal of Physics: Conference Series*, *795*(1), 012016. doi:10.1088/1742-6596/795/1/012016

Son, D., Lee, J., Qiao, S., Ghaffari, R., Kim, J., Lee, J. E., ... Yang, S. (2014). Multifunctional wearable devices for diagnosis and therapy of movement disorders. *Nature Nanotechnology*, *9*(5), 397–404. doi:10.1038/nnano.2014.38 PMID:24681776

Spencer, B. F. Jr, Ruiz-Sandoval, M., & Kurata, N. (2004, August). Smart sensing technology for structural health monitoring. *Proceedings of the 13th World Conference on Earthquake Engineering*.

Sreekanth, K. U., & Nitha, K. P. (2016). A study on health Care in Internet of Things. *International Journal on Recent and Innovation Trends in Computing and Communication*, *4*(2), 44–47.

Sundaram, P. (2013). Patient monitoring system using android technology. *International Journal of Computer Science and Mobile Computing*, *2*(5), 191–201.

Ufoaroh, S. U., Oranugo, C. O., & Uchechukwu, M. E. (2015). Heartbeat monitoring and alert system using GSM technology. *International Journal of Engineering Research and General Science, 3*(4), 26–34.

Zanella, A., Bui, N., Castellani, A., Vangelista, L., & Zorzi, M. (2014). Internet of things for smart cities. *IEEE Internet of Things Journal, 1*(1), 22-32.

# Chapter 2
# Smart Healthcare

**R. Rajkumar**
*VIT University, India*

## ABSTRACT

*Internet of things is a revolutionary domain, when we use it for the wellness of people in a smart way. As of now, the cost to implement IoT-enabled services is very high. So, this chapter introduces a cost effective and a reliable system to monitor patients at home and in hospitals with the help of IoT. The monitored details of a person can be drawn at any time with the help of an android app, which can produce output at real-time. The processed data are stored in the UBIDOTS cloud server, and the patients' needs can be met in time as well lives saved during critical cases with the help of the system proposed in this chapter.*

## INTRODUCTION

A Computer system that controls and accomplishes all the data in the hospital database to provide effective health care is called hospital information system (HIS). These health care systems have been existing since 1960s and have developed over time with better facilities. When they were in early stages, those systems didn't provide solution faster when applied in real time, but now system provide solution faster and reliable. The introduction of HIS made billing and inventor easier for the staff. But, now all the hospitals want to integrate the clinical, financial and other reports together to make the entire process a closed loop. This not only benefits the staff and patients to track the details but also make the discharge process also easier and faster.

DOI: 10.4018/978-1-5225-5036-5.ch002

Modern healthcare system requires integration of various departments which can be categorized as Core modules, supporting modules and Enterprise modules. Code Module includes Patient Accounts, Diagnostic Imaging, Radiology, Oncology, Ophthalmology, Orthopedics, Otolaryngology, etc. Supporting Modules includes Blood Bank, Elderly services, General Services, Patient Services, Purchasing & Supplies, Therapy, Pharmacy and Health & Safety. Enterprise management include Finance and Human Resources. These departments need to be integrated to retrieve patient details easily during emergencies and discharge.

Earlier there used to be many systems which provide the facility for managing the clinical records which are fixed at a place. It is quite complicated to get the information and make this data available at patient's bed side. The attendants for the patient have to physically go to the location and manually enter that data into those PC's which can lead to redundancy, data misplacement and errors in recording the data. This leads to considerable amount of wastage of time in moving to those storage PCs and also the cost afforded is comparatively high. Now-a-days, almost all the European countries are already having local area network (LAN) and wide area network (WAN). This eliminates the conventional process of treatment for the patient.

When maintaining the clinical record, many other details should be continuously monitored like whether the hospital bills are clear as per the due date which is to be collected from the administration department and also the availability of all the essential drugs to be supplied for the patient should be checked in advance from the logistics department. All this patient data must be exchanged between doctor and nurse and always they should be synchronized accordingly.

This problem can be handled by having mobile computers which are connected to a central database through the wireless connection. The servers will be connected to the wired or wireless LAN with hospital systems. The appropriate alert messages can be triggered by the server if the drugs are out of stock or if the patient needs to be attended by the doctor at the hour. Many systems are already being developed using wireless technologies by provided personal digital assistant (PDA) in hand.

As the world is moving with science and its latest inventions, there is a need for everyone to revolutionize the field of healthcare with them. The healthcare is a lifesaving division and is very much needed by any individual at any time. So, there should be a mandatory improvement that should be done to make healthcare more reliable and cost effective. Internet ia a big boon for the development of *iot* in all fields as the number of internet users have increased in a tremendous rate. This makes the *iot* to come into play. Which will make life easy for every individual? Assume a life where things get initiated on its own, where you need not have to produce a reminder or think about it. i.e If the milk in the refrigerator is going to be out of stock in another few hours. The *iot* enabled refrigerator will automatically order for milk to a nearby super market through *sms* or email or through an e-shopping site. Consider a hospital where there is a lack of staffs the patients admitted in the hospital should be given proper care or medication like i.e saline, pills, syringes etc in most needed time. If the hospital is *iot* enabled, one means the patient relatives can take care of them because *iot* enabled in a hospital will initiate all the needs of the patient on time. So, this can be done in a systematic way.

Imagine an industrialization place where any kind of accidents may occur at any time like i.e. fire, smoke, sound etc. when the place is enabled with *iot* sensors can be initiated in all places through the industry and the accidents that is going to happen can be sort out beforehand. And the employees can be guided in a safe path to leave the place of accident with the help of *iot* instructions. An automated home where it captures images of all the people by cameras before they make entry to the home and alerts the admin if a stranger is detected. We can set burglar alarms to some places or gadgets like wardrobe etc. where precious and expensive things are kept. When there is a disturbance it will alarm and makes call automatically to the admin. This model can be set in banks and other institutions which provide security to public property. In the field of security by using some robots in the places where no person can reach. Many fraudulent and the evil forces rising against the nation can be found by using *iot*.

## Existing Work

In (Borodin, Zavyalova, Zaharov, & Yamushev, 2015) *ecg* and heart rate are monitored with the help of a app where the data's are stored in local storage and in cloud memory and can keep an eye on the patients' health progress. In (La, Kim, & Kim, 2015) we are monitoring diseases like hypertension, diabetes and *ecg* they are integrated in a sensor kit. The outcome values can be monitored on desktop. The introduction of a smart gateway where the data from the sensors are stored in the cloud *db* and user *db*. All the data are received from the sensors through wireless medium (Catarinucci, De Donno, Mainetti, Palano, Patrono, Stefanizzi, & Tarricone, 2015). Data's are stored in the cloud server through internet web clients can use smartphones and laptops to see the data of the accelerometer and *ecg* are made in this paper (Rahmani, Thanigaivelan, Gia, Granados, Negash, Liljeberg, & Tenhunen, 2015) but a power efficient one. With the help of *phinet*as the cloud service we integrate all the actions performed values from the sensors like accelerometer, temperature, *ecg* and air flow sensor can be visualizing by healthcare professionals (Seales, Do, Belyi, & Kumar, 2015]. BSN body sensor network where we monitor details of sensor like *eeg*, *emg*, Blood Pressure, Motion Detection, *ecg* and temperature with the help of internet to the *bsn* care server where the local physicians and emergency team will take care of them (Gope, & Hwang, 2016]. In (Chiuchisan, Chiuchisan, & Dimian, 2015) we monitor the blood pressure, pulse and oxygen, electrocardiogram, patient position and body temperature with the help of the microcontroller to the clients like doctor, family, friends and emergency team with the help of internet and also as implementation of mobile app. In (Serdaroglu, Uslu, & Baydere, 2015) activity recognition has been implemented for the patients to monitor whether the elderly persons are taking pills or the medications at the right time prescribed by the physicians with the help of *rfid* tag and reader. If the person is inactive during the prescribed time an alert will be sent to the admin. Electrocardiogram is used to sense the health of the patient and monitor it updates the values at regular intervals to the website. Forwarding the values as a message to the doctor if any abnormal value is found and also turning on the buzzer (Gupta, Patchava, & Menezes, 2015]. The author proposes a system which does indoor, outdoor, emergency rescue and remote monitoring for dementia patients by locating the patient's position. The indoor system keeps a check on dementia patient and sends a notification to the neighborhoods. This uses a near field communication network whereas the outdoor monitoring uses a GSM network. The purpose of this paper is to integrate radio frequency identification (RFID) with GPS (global positioning system), Global system for mobile communication (GSM) and Global information system(GIS) to monitor and collect the status information from them. The architecture consists of a web server, a database and message controller server and a health GIS-server.

- **Indoor Monitoring:** It makes a call to the call center automatically when the elder person leaves home alone without notice. This message will be immediately received by the patient's care takers.

- **Outdoor Monitoring:** A pre-set outdoor area can be chosen, so that it constants checks if the patient is in that particular area. If the patient leaves the area, an alarm will be sent to the family through GSM network.
- **Emergency Rescue:** The patient who is in emergency situation can signal the call Centre so that the geo position and profile details will be transmitted to the care takers. Remote monitoring: To get a single or periodic location report of the patient care takers can authenticate and use the system to track the patient.

The longitude and latitude co-ordinates of the patient received by the call center are converted to street map location using GPS and GIS parser and this information is combined with the personal profile information for a complete report. Each time a TIP (Tracing Information Packet) is generated and stored in the database. There will also be GPSlog, GISlog and Message log tables to store all up to date information of each segment of transmission process.

To monitor the patient constantly, sensors affixed to the body parts are used. To sense, process and transmit the sensor data use of RFID reader, a microprocessor and GSM communication module is beneficial. GSM satellite location module provides location information of the patient. The Short Message Controller receives the latest GPS data, H-GIS produces two GIS images with different resolutions to display appropriate GIS (Lin, Chiu, Hsiao, Lee, & Tsai, 2006).

This system delivers a laid-back monitoring scheme to solve the health problems in out fast-paced world. Difficulties in searching for a hospital and travelling in traffic are the major problem that needed to be addressed. The telemedicine system for patient monitoring allows the device to collect the vital signal records, therapy and medication records and provide treatment for the patient. The Solution for telemedicine comprises a stable GSM or satellite communication which provides more flexibility in offering service. Since, a mobile phone has become a necessary product, it can be connected to electro medic devices to transfer the patient data. These data are transported through serial port using an RS232 Interface.

The architecture comprises of a server along with data storage which acquires the data through TCP/UDP. The electomedic device collect vital signals such as ECG, heart rate, Blood pressure, SPO2, respiration rate and temperature and sends to mobile phone through RS232 Interface. These signals are converted into packets and the sent to server through internet. Since the connectivity might become a problem, the communication protocol has to be defined in the module. In this paper, Agilent A3 patient monitor is used in implementation. JAVA MIDP (Mobile Information Device Profile) is used for simple user interface as it contains commands.

The data in the server needs to be retrieved and analyzed faster. Therefore, a distributed system was developed under JAVA technology. Their implementation provided options to visualize the list and export them if needed. The system's transmission rate was 0.6sec per packet for an ECG signal and 2sec for heartrate. The loss in the data signals were handled by Error correction method CRC resulting in a reliable transfer and retrieval of data. This project was aimed to be an alternative to elderly and handicapped patients to assist their health from a distance and also reduced the travelling cost and time.

*Figure 1. M-Smart Healthcare Architecture*

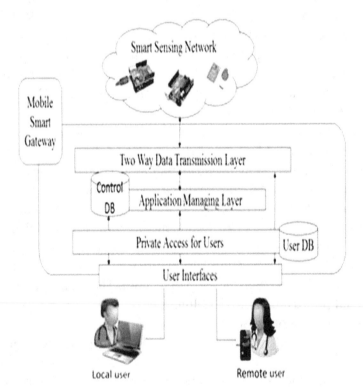

## System Architecture

In this proposed architecture in Figure 1 we introduce sensors like heartbeat, alcohol, temperature and positioning sensor. It can be used in homes and in hospitals we connect all the sensors to the Arduino microcontroller in a wireless way. So, the data that is produced at the sensors some distance away from the Arduino microcontroller can receive it. The heart beat sensor is used to measure the heart rate of a person. It can be used in both homes and in hospitals. The alcohol sensor is used in hospitals and not in homes when a person is found to be consumed with liquor the treatment will be temporarily stopped for the person in any emergency case. As the alcohol inside the patient's body will become toxic if any medication is given. Temperature sensor is used to determine a room's temperature it will be helpful during dramatic climatic changes if the person does not have a sense of feeling to express whether they have a sultry feeling when there is an increase in temperature and shivering due to low in temperature. The position sensor will produce output according to the movement of the patients. If the patient moves to the left side a range of values is produced in the x, y and z axis. If the patient turns to the right another set of x, y and z axis values will be produced. Similarly, for the patients lying and standing position. In Figure 2 All the sensors will work only if the person has a valid *rfid* tag that has been assigned to the patient beforehand. Patient and family are the users of the healthcare system where the patient health is tracked by the sensor attached through the wireless portable phone which has an installed Application to send the Protected Health Information details known as PHI.

The Patient Application is installed in electronic device such as smartphone, PDA or a secure wearable device. The device lets the family of the patient know the status of the patient and provides alert messages to the concerned persons of the patient in case of emergency based on the priority of the alert message and also it redirects the alert if the alert situation is not attended within a specific time period.

The ECG monitor used in the proposed model is DARDIOCARE which is a wireless wearable device. The device seamlessly fits the patient and provides accurate monitoring of the heart activity in daily basis. The data can be remotely accessed from the device and provides doctor/ physician accurate information. It not only measures heartrate but also body temperature, stress level, respiratory rate and tracks the activity of the patient.

*Figure 2. Microcontroller connected RFID and Sensors*

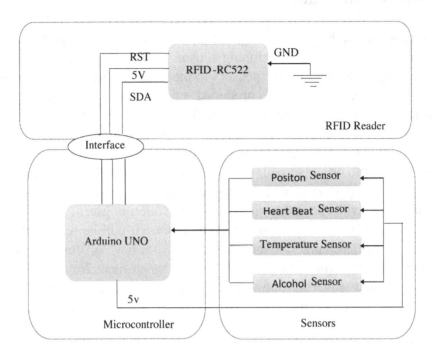

If it is a valid tag the *uid* will be produced and the arduino microcontroller in Figure 3 will start reading the values. If it is not a valid one, it will ignore reading the values. The data's read from the sensors are sent to the internet by means of ethernet shield. The ethernet shield is installed in such a way that it transmits data to the *ubidots* cloud server with the help of the internet. An account has been created in *ubidots* for the data from the sensors to get stored. The data gets updated at once it is uploaded by the sensors. Now it is possible for the users to access the *ubidots* to monitor details of a person in real-time. The data from the sensors are classified beforehand as healthy and critical data all the normal values will be stored in in a local storage i.e *sd* card and all the critical values will be stored in *ubidots* cloud server in order to save data. Once the critical data gets allocated into the memory of the *ubidots*. It will take action on it by automatically initiating text message and e-mail to the recipients like relatives, family and emergency team. This whole system can be viewed or monitored by means of an android app. Where it requires an android supported smartphone can track information remotely when away from the patients.

*Figure 3. Bread Board interface between Arduino and Sensors*

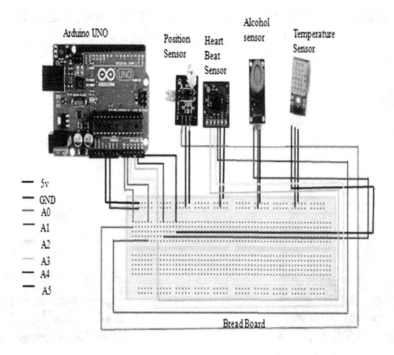

## Implementation

The following algorithm has been proposed in the following:

- Add the sensor modules.
- Let the sensors heartbeat, temperature, alcohol and accelerometer communicate with the Arduino.
- Get the input values from the sensors.
- Update the values to the *ubidots* cloud server.
- If any of the values not in range send intimation to the recipients through *sms* or e-mail.
- If the values are normal continue monitoring.

In the app version, we can send appointments to the doctor for checkup and the doctor has to approve according to his schedule and an acknowledgement will be sent on all successful approval as in Figure 4.

*Figure 4. Results of Mobile Monitoring App*

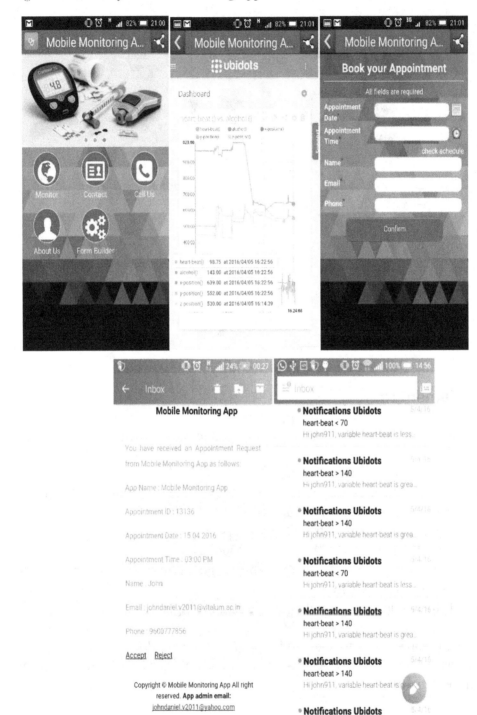

*Table 1. Comparative Approach*

| Reference Work | Technologies | | | Services Provided | | | |
|---|---|---|---|---|---|---|---|
| | RFID | WSN | Mobile | Patient Tracking | Staff Tracking | Remote Patient Monitoring | Alert Notification |
| 1 | | P | P | P | | P | |
| 2 | | | P | | | P | P |
| 3 | | | | P | P | | |
| 4 | | P | | P | | P | |
| 5 | | P | P | | | P | |
| 6 | | P | P | P | | | P |
| 7 | | P | | | | P | |
| 8 | P | P | P | P | | P | P |
| 9 | | P | | P | | P | P |
| Proposed System | P | P | P | P | P | P | P |

# CONCLUSION

We have proposed a system which is cost effective and reliable collects data wirelessly and stores data both in local memory like *sd* card and in cloud server. We have implemented to conserve data and a mobile application to know the wellness condition of the patient. The normal healthy data are stored in the *sd* card and the critical data are sent to the *ubidots* cloud server. Where data will be validated automatically and intimation will be sent to all reciepients like family, relative and emergency team. This proposed system will be very useful to save their life in time before some tragedy happens.

As a future work, we can concentrate on data mining part because to reduce the volume of data that is stored. The patient's medical data will be compared the existing patient's database the diseases at the initial stage can be found out. Regarding the issue and a proper precautionary step can be made before something that risks the patient life happens and also, we can work on availing more security to the proposed system as the data transferred are confidential.

# REFERENCES

Borodin, A., Zavyalova, Y., Zaharov, A., & Yamushev, I. (2015, April). Architectural approach to the multisource health monitoring application design. In *Open Innovations Association (FRUCT), 2015 17th Conference of* (pp. 16-21). IEEE. 10.1109/FRUCT.2015.7117965

Catarinucci, L., De Donno, D., Mainetti, L., Palano, L., Patrono, L., Stefanizzi, M. L., & Tarricone, L. (2015). An IoT-aware architecture for smart healthcare systems. *IEEE Internet of Things Journal*, 2(6), 515–526. doi:10.1109/JIOT.2015.2417684

Chiuchisan, I., Chiuchisan, I., & Dimian, M. (2015, October). Internet of Things for e-Health: An approach to medical applications. In *Computational Intelligence for Multimedia Understanding (IWCIM), 2015 International Workshop on* (pp. 1-5). IEEE.

Gope, P., & Hwang, T. (2016). BSN-Care: A secure IoT-based modern healthcare system using body sensor network. *IEEE Sensors Journal*, 16(5), 1368–1376. doi:10.1109/JSEN.2015.2502401

Gupta, M. S. D., Patchava, V., & Menezes, V. (2015, October). Healthcare based on IoT using Raspberry Pi. In *Green Computing and Internet of Things (ICGCIoT), 2015 International Conference on* (pp. 796-799). IEEE. 10.1109/ICGCIoT.2015.7380571

La, H. J., Kim, M. K., & Kim, S. D. (2015, June). A Personal Healthcare System with Inference-as-a-Service. In *Services Computing (SCC), 2015 IEEE International Conference on* (pp. 249-255). IEEE. 10.1109/SCC.2015.42

Lin, C. C., Chiu, M. J., Hsiao, C. C., Lee, R. G., & Tsai, Y. S. (2006). Wireless health care service system for elderly with dementia. *IEEE Transactions on Information Technology in Biomedicine*, 10(4), 696–704. doi:10.1109/TITB.2006.874196 PMID:17044403

Rahmani, A. M., Thanigaivelan, N. K., Gia, T. N., Granados, J., Negash, B., Liljeberg, P., & Tenhunen, H. (2015, January). Smart e-health gateway: Bringing intelligence to internet-of-things based ubiquitous healthcare systems. In *Consumer Communications and Networking Conference (CCNC), 2015 12th Annual IEEE* (pp. 826-834). IEEE. 10.1109/CCNC.2015.7158084

Seales, C., Do, T., Belyi, E., & Kumar, S. (2015, June). PHINet: A Plug-n-Play Content-centric Testbed Framework for Health-Internet of Things. In *Mobile Services (MS), 2015 IEEE International Conference on* (pp. 368-375). IEEE. 10.1109/MobServ.2015.57

Serdaroglu, K., Uslu, G., & Baydere, S. (2015, October). Medication intake adherence with real time activity recognition on IoT. In *Wireless and Mobile Computing, Networking and Communications (WiMob), 2015 IEEE 11th International Conference on* (pp. 230-237). IEEE. 10.1109/WiMOB.2015.7347966

# Chapter 3
# Smart Healthcare Administration Over Cloud

**Govinda K.**
*VIT University, India*

**S. Ramasubbareddy**
*VIT University, India*

## ABSTRACT

*Cloud computing is an emerging technology that is expected to support internet-scale critical applications, which could be essential to the healthcare sector. Its scalability, resilience, adaptability, connectivity, cost reduction, and high-performance features have high potential to lift the efficiency and quality of healthcare. With the widespread application of healthcare information and communication technology, constructing a stable and sustainable data sharing circumstance has attracted rapidly growing attention in both academic research area and the healthcare industry. Cloud computing is one of long dreamed visions of healthcare cloud (HC), which matches the need of healthcare workers, information sharing directly to various health providers over the internet, regardless of their location and the amount of data. This chapter proposes a cloud model for health information sharing and integration in HC and looks into the arising challenges in healthcare.*

DOI: 10.4018/978-1-5225-5036-5.ch003

# INTRODUCTION

With the development in healthcare and economic fields, more number of medical records are generated. There is an urgent need and demand to improve the levels and standards of modern health-care records management by using innovative technology. The objective of this paper is to introduce the concept of Cloud Computing and discuss the challenges of applying Healthcare Cloud (HC) to improve the Health Information Science research. With the new concept of Cloud Computing emerging in recent years, more and more interests have been sparked from a variety organizations and individual users, as they increasingly intend to take advantage of web applications to share a huge amount of public and private data and information in a more affordable way and reliable IT architecture.

More specifically, the medical and health information system based on the cloud computing is desired, in order to realize the sharing of medical data and health information, coordination of clinical service, along with the effective and cost-containment clinical information system infrastructure via the implementation of a distributed and high-integrated platform.

Mobile devices are growing in terms of utilization in our daily life to voice conversations and video chatting with others. Especially the smart phones became an important tool in our daily activities in e-commerce, IT industries. Even though mobile device is capable of enough to handle high end applications but still suffering with limited resources such as short battery lifetime, storage and processor. These changes help users to make environment where all devices share resources to run application efficiently.

The conventional computing only deals with the compute and process computation tasks. The modern technologies got birth to satisfy user requirements; Big data, networking, cloud computing, fog computing, mobile cloud computing, IOT, the user will always require modern infrastructure to achieve increasing demand on both mobility and connectivity (Goswami, 2013). Among many technologies mobile cloud computing became a popular model (Zimmerman, 1999). Mobile computing allows many devices interacting with other mobile devices through network technologies (Wi-Fi and 4G). The mobile devices have many advantages like portability and mobility features. The mobile computing is integrated with cloud computing technology in order to form new technology called as MCC (Bahwaireth, Lo'ai, Tawalbeh, Benkhelifa, Jararweh, & Tawalbeh, 2016). The MCC can overcome the limitations of mobile device. In the case of implementing real MCC model, we have to take into account few challenges which cause troubles while establishing MCC environment. Mobile devices are limited by storage, battery lifetime, processing, and video streaming, augmented reality application. We should consider another important challenge in the mobility of device are moving from one network environment to another network environment. This affects quality of performance and connectivity with remote cloud (Qi, & Gani, 2012). The MCC can avoid limitations of mobile device by offloading computational task into remote cloud which requires more processing power locally. In result the remote cloud will process it with less power consumption (Benkhelifa, Welsh, Tawalbeh, Jaraweh, & Basalamah, 2015). MCC is considered as new trend among many new technologies in coming years. Generally the mobile devices connecting to cloud computing via various network technologies such as 3G and 4G. These technologies cause high cost, limited bandwidth and connectivity problems as shown in Figure 1. The important issue is nothing but security. Providing security to data from attackers over wire or wireless channel (Moh'd, Aslam, Marzi, & Tawalbeh, 2010) is a big challenge in both cloud and mobile cloud computing. The user always expects his data need to be safe and not to be affected by attackers (Tawalbeh, & Eardley, 2010]. There are many encryption techniques to protect data from attackers (Tawalbeh, Jararweh, & Mohammad, 2012; Tawalbeh, Tenca, Park, & Koc, 2004].

Since health informatics seek new ways of driving health information science research forward, for example, international research collaboration, growing demands are now placed on computer networks to provide hardware and software resources and pave a new avenue to share sensitive and private medical data from different geographic locations. This new model of service (Cloud Computing) offers tremendous opportunities for the collaborative health information science research purpose; unfortunately, it has also introduced a set of new and unfamiliar challenges, such as lack of interoperability, standardization, privacy, network security and culture resistance. In this paper, we will identify the challenges of applying healthcare cloud in the health information research and discuss potential approaches to conquer those barriers, such as audit, disaster recovery, legal, regulatory and compliance.

Finally, the paper will focus on the security of Cloud Computing applied in the health information science research. Research on the various security issues surrounding healthcare information systems has been heated over the last few years.

# LITERATURE REVIEW

The advent of cloud computing in recent years has increased a lot of interests from different stakeholders, business organizations, institutions and government agencies. The growing interest is fueled by the promised new economic model of cloud computing which brings a change from heavy IT infrastructure invest for limiting resources that are internally managed and owned to pay per use for IT service owned by a service provider. Cloud computing paves a new avenue to deliver enterprise IT. As all major disruptive changes in technology and Internet revolution, it represents an innovative democratized of Web computing. Cloud computing not only upgrade the business models and the way IT infrastructure is being consumed, but also the underlying architecture of how we develop, deploy, run and deliver applications.

The researches have been putting lot of efforts across the world for improving Mobile cloud computing. The users require numerous application in mobile device, each of these application require data exchange and receive as well as require lot of processing power. This paper (D. Huang, 2011), describes how the mobile computing is formed from both mobile computing and cloud computing. The author also discussed about challenges, scope of MCC and development. The sensors in network technology inspired lot of researchers in world to collect data from different useful aspects of life in clouding military, hospital, IT organization, education institutions, and crowd management (Lo'ai, & Bakhader, 2016). The huge amount of data will be generated every day that data need to be stored efficiently all that data has to be stored in cloud server for storage and processing (Lo'ai, & Bakhader, 2016) . In paper (Miettinen, & Nurminen, 2010), the author has analyzed main factors which cause more power consumption in mobile devices while using remote cloud. This provided an example on how to save energy between mobile device and remote cloud. They have discussed main characteristics of modern mobile device. The jobs from users can be schedule among VMs inside cloudlet was discussed in (Shiraz& Gani, 2012). The key metrics are overhead of VM life cycle, scheduling of VM, job allocation to VM. The author in (Lo'ai, & Bakhader, 2016) has discussed importance of scheduling of VMs in cloud environment in order to reduce execution time by using Cloudsim cloud environment tool. This paper proposes architecture was fine grained cloudlet to manage all applications inside cloudlet. The cloudlet can be chosen dynamically not like previous model. The cloudlet is fixed near wireless access point. In this paper (Jararweh, Ababneh, Khreishah,

& Dosari, 2014], the author had proposed mobile cloud computing model which is different from other previous published model in terms of scalability features. These paper experimental results have covered intended numbers of cloudlets available in covered area. The mobile device is known to acquire more power while running excessive applications. The author is motivated by the fact that optimizing power is important in MCC. In this paper (Al-Ayyoub, Jararweh, Lo'ai, Tawalbeh, Benkhelifa & Basalamah, 2015), the author had produced mathematical model to optimize power consumption in MCC. The author in (Tawalbeh, & Eardley, 2016), had conducted experiment on mobile device by analyzing each and every component and cloudlet each component participation in total power consumption.

## Definition of Cloud Computing

Mell and Grance (2010) give a definition of cloud computing that is a model for enabling convenient, on-demand network access to a shared pool of configurable computing resource that can be rapidly provisioned and released with minimal management effort or service-provider interaction. We have already seen similar more limited applications for years, such as Google Docs or Gmail. Nevertheless, cloud computing is different from traditional systems (Mell, & Grance, 2010). Armbrust et al. introduce that cloud computing offers a wide range of computing sources on demand anywhere and anytime; eliminates an up-front commitment by cloud users; allows users to pay for use of computing resources on a short-term basis as needed and has higher utilization by multiplexing of workloads from various organizations. Cloud computing includes three models: (1) Software as a Service (SaaS): the applications (e.g. EHRs) are hosted by a cloud service provider and made available to customers over a network, typically the Internet;

(2) Platform as a Service (PaaS): the development tools (such as OS system) are hosted in the cloud and accessed through a browser (e.g. Microsoft Azure); (3) Infrastructure as a Service (IaaS): the cloud user outsources the equipment used to support operations, including storage, hardware, servers and networking components. The cloud service provider owns the equipment and is responsible for housing, running and maintaining it (Armbrust, Fox, Griffith, Joseph, Katz, Konwinski, ... & Zaharia, 2010). In the clinical environment, healthcare providers are able to remotely access the corporate Intranet via a local Internet service provider, since they have the option to have an ISDN line installed to their home or hospital linking with Cloud.

## Application of Cloud Computing in Healthcare

The majority of physicians in healthcare do not always have the information they require when they need to rapidly make patient-care decisions, and patients often have to carry a paper record of their health history information with them from visit to visit. To address the problems, IBM and Active Health Management collaborate to create a cloud computing technology-based Collaborative Care solution that gives physicians and patients access to the information they need to improve the overall quality of care, without the need to invest in new infrastructure (Guo, Kuo, & Sahama, 2012). IBM facilitated American Occupational Network and HyGen Pharmaceuticals to improve patient care by digitizing health records and streamlining their business operations using cloud-based software from IBM MedTrak systems, Inc. and The System House, Inc. Their technology handles various tasks as a cloud service through the internet instead of developing, purchasing and maintaining technology onsite (Guo, Kuo, & Sahama, 2012). Acumen solution's cloud computing CRM and project management system were selected by the U.S. Department of Health & Human Services' office of the National.

Coordinator for Health IT to manage the selection and implementation of EHR systems across the country. The software will enable regional extension centers to manage interactions with medical providers related to the selection and implementation of an EHR system. Sharp Community Medical Group in San Diego will be using the collaborative.

Care solution to change the way physicians and nurse's access information throughout the hospital group's multiple electronic medical record systems to apply advanced analytical and clinical decision support to help give doctors better insight and work more closely with patient care teams (Guo, Kuo, & Sahama, 2012). One of similar example of applying cloud service in the healthcare area is the architecture of the hospital file management system (HFMS). A HFMS cluster contains a master server and multiple blocks of servers by multiple client access.

## PROPOSED METHOD

I have presented an overview of the security challenges in the healthcare information sharing, and Different security concerns related to threats and vulnerabilities are analyzed. Here, we propose ways of alleviating these

*Figure 1. Overview of HFMS*

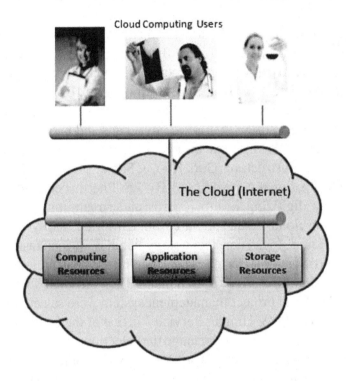

*Figure 2. Proposed architecture of smart healthcare over cloud*

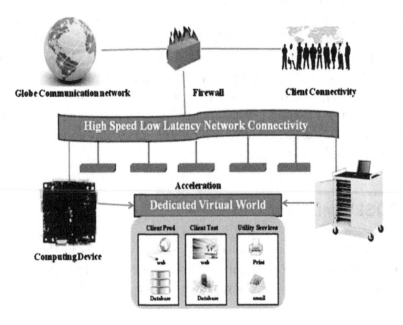

barriers. There are steps we can take to reduce the risk that an EHR system will be hacked:

- Keep the EHR on a segregated network, if possible. Shelter the EHR from the rest of the network infrastructure. Otherwise it's very easy for a provider's practice management system or mobile or medical device to pass on a virus or other infiltration to the EHR system.
- Check for vulnerabilities. Run risk assessments and conduct audits. Correct weaknesses discovered.
- Consider buying and running a data loss prevention software program, which runs on the perimeter server.
- Apply security patches to internet applications that are connected to the EHR systems, such as internet explorer, java and adobe acrobat.
- Make sure that the firewalls are installed properly, and that the antivirus programs are operational. Hackers are looking for easy access into computer networks. Don't make the EHR system that easy a target.
- Comply with objective, specific measures, such as those recommended by the National Institute of Standards and Technology or HITRUST, so you can defend the adequacy of the safeguards you took to protect patient information.
- Make sure that the EHR and health IT vendor contracts support off-the-shelf antivirus software.
- Designate who within the organization is responsible for maintaining the integrity of the system.
- Clearly delineate with the EHR/Health IT vendor who will be responsible for security patches. Don't assume that the vendor will do it; many vendors don't.
- Make sure that any medical software you're working with runs without "super user" rights. This makes it harder for a hacker to gain access to the records.

## SECURITY MEASURES

Cloud security architecture is effective only if the correct defensive implementations are in place. An efficient cloud security architecture should recognize the issues that will arise with security management. The security management addresses these issues with security controls. These controls are put in place to safeguard any weaknesses in the system and reduce the effect of an attack. While there are many types of controls behind a cloud security architecture, they can usually be found in one of the following categories:

- **Deterrent Controls:** These controls are intended to reduce attacks on a cloud system. Much like a warning sign on a fence or a property, deterrent controls typically reduce the threat level by informing potential attackers that there will be adverse consequences for them if they proceed. (Some consider them a subset of preventive controls.)
- **Preventive Controls:** Preventive controls strengthen the system against incidents, generally by reducing if not actually eliminating vulnerabilities. Strong authentication of cloud users, for instance, makes it less likely that unauthorized users can access cloud systems, and more likely that cloud users are positively identified.

## Physical Security

Cloud service providers physically secure the IT hardware (servers, routers, cables etc.) against unauthorized access, interference, theft, fires, floods etc. and ensure that essential supplies (such as electricity) are sufficiently robust to minimize the possibility of disruption. This is normally achieved by serving cloud applications from 'world-class' (i.e. professionally specified, designed, constructed, managed, monitored and maintained) data centers.

## Personnel Security

Various information security concerns relating to the IT and other professionals associated with cloud services are typically handled through pre-, para- and post-employment activities such as security screening potential recruits, security awareness and training programs, proactive

## Privacy

Providers ensure that all critical data (credit card numbers, for example) are masked or encrypted and that only authorized users have access to data in its entirety. Moreover, digital identities and credentials must be protected as should any data that the provider collects or produces about customer activity in the cloud.

## ENCRYPTION MEASURES

## Attribute-Based Encryption Algorithm

### Cipher Text-Policy ABE (CP-ABE)

In the CP-ABE, the encryptor controls access strategy, as the strategy gets more complex, the design of system public key becomes more complex, and the security of the system is proved to be more difficult. The main research work of CP-ABE is focused on the design of the access structure.

In the KP-ABE, attribute sets are used to explain the encrypted texts and the private keys with the specified encrypted texts that users will have the left to decrypt.

### Fully Homomorphic Encryption (FHE)

Fully Homomorphic encryption allows straightforward computations on encrypted information, and also allows computing sum and product for the encrypted data without decryption.

### Searchable Encryption (SE)

Searchable Encryption is a cryptographic primitive which offers secure search functions over encrypted data. In order to improve search efficiency, an SE solution generally builds keyword indexes to securely perform user queries. Existing SE schemes can be classified into two categories: SE based on secret-key cryptography and SE based on public-key cryptography.

## THE CLOUDLET USES IN E-HEALTH SYATEMS

In E-healthcare systems, the cloud computing and cloudlet technologies are required. The cloudlet technology is available to analyze patient records and also process, extract recommended features from patient database. In this system, we discussed the state of art on healthcare systems in cloud computing the application growth on healthcare is growing day by day. Also this application requires lot of computation and communication resources. The application requires access huge amount of data from organizations within and outside of the boundaries. The data pattern is typically dynamic. It is only support granularity interaction. In cloud environment (Mehmood, Faisal, & Altowaijri, 2015), the future application will have to support heterogeneous platform inside (or) outside organization (Macias, & Thomas, 2011). There is no wonder to say that the advantages of cloud computing can be helpful for the organization including healthcare systems. The healthcare organization depends on cloud environment for processing and storage of huge amount of data. Another important challenge is risk management. The cost of maintained health data is stored in cloud (Lo'ai, Bakhader, Mehmood, & Song, 2016) because of sensitivity of health data. The cost of health maintained data and also provide privacy and security laws is gradually growing. Taking decision for storing of data of healthcare and other organizations into cloud required lot of confidence. In this paper (Mehmood, Faisal, & Altowaijri, 2015), the author had proposed transport load and capacity sharing. The healthcare systems in smart city meeting demands by adapting cloud computing. The cloud computing is beneficial because distribution of cloudlet across world. The study on grid computing shared poor accessing remotely. How it useful in healthcare applications deployment is presented (Altowaijri, Mehmood, & Williams, 2010). Though the paper is focused on grid computing, it also suits for cloud computing technology. Multiple organizations and application scenarios for deployment of grid computing based on different classes of organization as well as various types of applications. The requirements of healthcare system is identified and analyzed based on result of iteration in terms of throughput. This platform identifies the computational and communicational requirements of healthcare system application. This analysis is important because the network traffic connecting health care system is dominated by analytical applications which require zero network latencies. The individual request is not heavy in terms of data but causes heavy traffic in feature communication. The cloudlet concept can be applied on this communication and computation concept in order to analyze the performance of cloud computing health care application. In this paper (Council, 2016), the author had discussed adaption of cloud solutions in healthcare systems in order to make health service provider move forward. Also, discussed privacy, security, risk management and work flow challenges. There are many papers in cloud computing focused on health care applications including foundation for health care (IBM, 2016), impact of cloud computing on healthcare (Council, 2016).

## RESULTS

## Comparison Between Full Homomorphic and Attribute Based Encryption

See Figures 3-5.

## CONCLUSION

Little literature in the health information science research addresses the critical challenges and solutions of applying Cloud Computing. While the use of Cloud Computing continues to increase, legal concerns are also increasing. Although Cloud Computing providers may run afoul of the obstacles, we believe that over the long run providers will successfully navigate these challenges. By using Cloud Computing security framework, the collaborative parties can answer questions related to governance and best practice and determine whether the organization is capable of IT governance in the Cloud Computing applications.

*Figure 3. Comparison is based on time. Here the dark line refers to ABE method and light line belongs to FULL Homomorphic method. Hence ABE method is better.*

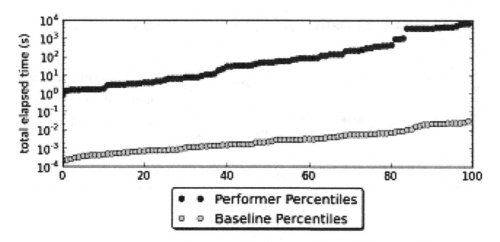

*Figure 4. Comparison based on efficiency (of computation); light line represents Full homomorphic and dark line ABE method. Hence ABE method is better.*

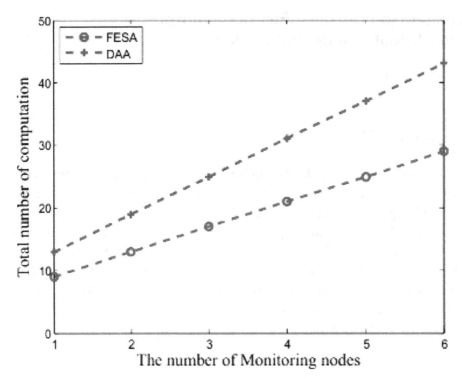

*Figure 5. Comparative Strength of ABE and RSA. Hence ABE method is better.*

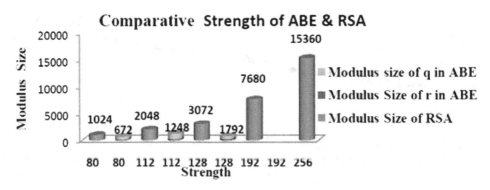

# REFERENCES

Al-Ayyoub, M., Jararweh, Y., Lo'ai, A., Tawalbeh, E., Benkhelifa & Basalamah. (2015). Power Optimization of Large Scale Mobile Cloud Computing Systems. In *Proceedings of the 3rd IEEE International conference on Future Internet of things and Cloud (Fi- Cloud)*. Rome, Italy: IEEE.

Altowaijri, S., Mehmood, R., & Williams, J. (2010, January). A quantitative model of grid systems performance in healthcare organisations. In *Intelligent Systems, Modelling and Simulation (ISMS), 2010 International Conference on* (pp. 431-436). IEEE. 10.1109/ISMS.2010.84

Ansi, I. (2003). TS 18308 health informatics-requirements for an electronic health record architecture. ISO.

Armbrust, M., Fox, A., Griffith, R., Joseph, A. D., Katz, R., Konwinski, A., ... Zaharia, M. (2010). A view of cloud computing. *Communications of the ACM, 53*(4), 50–58. doi:10.1145/1721654.1721672

Bahwaireth. (2016, June). Experimental Comparison of Simulation Tools for Efficient Cloud and Mobile Cloud Computing Applications. *EURASIP Journal on Information Security., 15*. doi:10.118613635-016-0039-y

Benkhelifa, E., Welsh, T., Tawalbeh, L., Jararweh, Y., & Basalamah, A. (2015). User profiling for energy optimisation in mobile cloud computing. *Procedia Computer Science, 52*, 1159–1165. doi:10.1016/j.procs.2015.05.151

Benkhelifa, E., Welsh, T., Tawalbeh, L., Khreishah, A., Jararweh, Y., & Al-Ayyoub, M. (2016, March). GA-Based Resource Augmentation Negotation for Energy-Optimised Mobile Ad-hoc Cloud. In *Mobile Cloud Computing, Services, and Engineering (MobileCloud), 2016 4th IEEE International Conference on* (pp. 110-116). IEEE. 10.1109/MobileCloud.2016.25

Council, C. S. C. (2012). *Impact of cloud computing on healthcare. Technical report*. Cloud Standards Customer Council.

Fox, A., Griffith, R., Joseph, A., Katz, R., Konwinski, A., Lee, G., ... Stoica, I. (2009). Above the clouds: A Berkeley view of cloud computing. Dept. Electrical Eng. and Comput. Sciences, University of California, Berkeley, Rep. UCB/EECS, 28(13), 2009.

Goswami. (2013). Mobile Computing. *Int. J. Adv. Res. Comput. Sci. Softw. Eng.*, 846–855.

Guo, Y., Kuo, M. H., & Sahama, T. (2012, December). Cloud computing for healthcare research information sharing. In *Cloud Computing Technology and Science (CloudCom), 2012 IEEE 4th International Conference on* (pp. 889-894). IEEE. 10.1109/CloudCom.2012.6427561

Huang, D., & ... (2011). Mobile cloud computing. *IEEE COMSOC Multimed. Commun. Tech. Comm. MMTC E-Lett.*, 6(10), 27–31.

IBM. (2011). *Cloud Computing: Building a New Foundation for Healthcare.* IBM Corporation. Available: https://www-05.ibm.com/de/healthcare/literature/cloud-newfoundation- for-hv.pdf

Jararweh, Y., Ababneh, F., Khreishah, A., & Dosari, F. (2014). Scalable cloudlet-based mobile computing model. *Procedia Computer Science, 34,* 434–441. doi:10.1016/j.procs.2014.07.051

Lo'ai, A. T., & Bakhader, W. (2016, August). A Mobile Cloud System for Different Useful Applications. In *Future Internet of Things and Cloud Workshops (FiCloudW), IEEE International Conference on* (pp. 295-298). IEEE.

Lo'ai, A. T., Bakhader, W., Mehmood, R., & Song, H. (2016, December). Cloudlet-based Mobile Cloud Computing for Healthcare Applications. In *Global Communications Conference (GLOBECOM)* (pp. 1-6). IEEE.

Lo'ai, A. T., Bakhader, W., Mehmood, R., & Song, H. (2016, December). Cloudlet-based Mobile Cloud Computing for Healthcare Applications. In *Global Communications Conference (GLOBECOM)* (pp. 1-6). IEEE.

Lo'ai, A. T., Bakheder, W., & Song, H. (2016, June). A mobile cloud computing model using the cloudlet scheme for big data applications. In *Connected Health: Applications, Systems and Engineering Technologies (CHASE), 2016 IEEE First International Conference on* (pp. 73-77). IEEE.

Macias, F., & Thomas, G. (2011). *Cloud Computing Advantages in the Public Sector: How Today's Government, Education, and Healthcare Organizations Are Benefiting from Cloud Computing Environments.* Retrieved from Cisco website: http://www. cisco. com/web/strategy/docs/c11-687784_cloud_omputing_wp. pdf

Mehmood, R., Faisal, M. A., & Altowaijri, S. (n.d.). Future Networked Healthcare Systems: A Review and Case Study. In Handbook Res. Redesigning Future Internet Archit. (pp. 564–590). Academic Press.

Mehmood, R., & Graham, G. (2015). Big data logistics: A health-care transport capacity sharing model. *Procedia Computer Science, 64*, 1107–1114. doi:10.1016/j.procs.2015.08.566

Mell, P., & Grance, T. (2010). *The NIST definition of cloud computing.* NIST.

Miettinen, A. P., & Nurminen, J. K. (2010). Energy Efficiency of Mobile Clients in Cloud Computing. *HotCloud, 10*, 4–4.

Moh'd, A., Aslam, N., Marzi, H., & Tawalbeh, L. A. (2010, July). Hardware implementations of secure hashing functions on FPGAs for WSNs. *Proceedings of the 3rd International Conference on the Applications of Digital Information and Web Technologies (ICADIWT.*

Mohammad, A., & Gutub, A. A. A. (2010). Efficient FPGA implementation of a programmable architecture for GF (p) elliptic curve crypto computations. *Journal of Signal Processing Systems for Signal, Image, and Video Technology, 59*(3), 233–244. doi:10.100711265-009-0376-x

Qi, H., & Gani, A. (2012, May). Research on mobile cloud computing: Review, trend and perspectives. In *Digital Information and Communication Technology and it's Applications (DICTAP), 2012 Second International Conference on* (pp. 195-202). IEEE.

Shiraz, M., & Gani, A. (2012, February). Mobile cloud computing: Critical analysis of application deployment in virtual machines. In *Proc. Int'l Conf. Information and Computer Networks (ICICN'12) (Vol. 27).* Academic Press.

Tawalbeh, L. A., Alassaf, N., Bakheder, W., & Tawalbeh, A. (2015, October). Resilience Mobile Cloud Computing: Features, Applications and Challenges. In *e-Learning (econf), 2015 Fifth International Conference on* (pp. 280-284). IEEE.

Tawalbeh, L. A., Jararweh, Y., & Mohammad, A. (2012). An integrated radix-4 modular divider/multiplier hardware architecture for cryptographic applications. *The International Arab Journal of Information Technology, 9*(3).

Tawalbeh, L. A., Tenca, Λ. F., Park, S., & Koc, C. K. (2004). A dualfield modular division algorithm and architecture for application specific hardware. In *Thirty-Eighth Asilomar Conference on Signals, Systems, and Computers* (pp. 483-487). IEEE Press.

Tawalbeh, M., Eardley, A., & Tawalbeh, L. (2016). Studying the energy consumption in mobile devices. *Procedia Computer Science*, *94*, 183–189. doi:10.1016/j.procs.2016.08.028

Zimmerman, J. B. (1999). Mobile computing: Characteristics, business benefits, and the mobile framework. *University of Maryland European Division-Bowie State*, *10*, 12.

Chapter 4

# A Survey of Mobile Computing Devices and Sensors in Healthcare Applications:
## Real-Time System Design

**Narayana Moorthi M.**
*VIT University, India*

**Manjula R.**
*VIT University, India*

## ABSTRACT

*Mobile devices are continuously improving, adding integrated sensors, which are of value to the healthcare industry. Sensor-enabled mobile phones collect data from patients, which is useful for doctors in providing immediate care and treatment. As smartphones become ubiquitous, their use as health monitors should become commonplace. This chapter surveys mobile computing devices and sensors in healthcare applications.*

## INTRODUCTION

The mobile devices (Kay, Santos, & Takane, 2011; Stankevich, E., Paramonov, I., & Timofeev, 2012) including personal digital assistant (PDA), smartphone, tablet computer, ultra-mobile PC, and wearable computers (Nosrati, Karimi, & Hasanvand, 2012; Ozkil, Fan, Dawids, Aanes, Kristensen, & Christensen, 2012; (Rajan, Spanias, Ranganath, Banavar, & Spanias) are useful for many

DOI: 10.4018/978-1-5225-5036-5.ch004

applications. They all work with different operating systems such as Symbian, Windows, Palm OS, BlackBerry, iOS, Android, and Bada. The cell phone is the combination of hardware and software. The following are few hardware devices. The Processor or microcontroller with different families, the key switches, LED, LCD, alarm or speaker, camera, microphone, battery or power supply and many sensors (Manjulal; Moorthi, & Vaideeswaran; Narayana Moorthi, & Manjula). Each family of microcontrollers has its own architecture and list of registers, memory management, addressing modes or methods, its own instruction set and assembly language.

The processor families include AVR, PIC, ARM and Intel 8051.

The 8051 is an 8-bit processor. The AVRs are also 8 bit, but some are 32 bit and ARMs are 32 bit, and are more powerful than 8 bit processors.

PIC is a family of Harvard architecture single chip microcontrollers made by Microchip Technology. The name PIC initially referred as Programmable Interface Controller. The 8051 is the very basic controller used for the simple applications, AVR and PIC are used to interface more advanced peripherals such as microSD card and RFID scanner etc and ARM is the most advanced controller family generally used for Real Time Applications.

The software includes the operating system modules from various vendors.

Introduction to Sensors: Sensor is a device which measures a physical quantity like temperature, pressure or force and converts it into an electrical signal which can be read by an instrument. These voltage or electrical signal is normally an Analog signal which can be converted to digital using ADC-Analog to digital converters.

Sensors on Android Phones: Access to the sensors on an Android phone is available through the class in the package of the android SDK (http://developer.android.com/sdk/).Not all sensors are present in all phones. Here the Table 1 is the list of sensors on the smartphone.

*Figure 1. Patient Care*

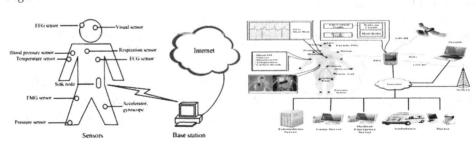

*Table 1. Summary of Sensors*

| Name of the Sensor | Purpose |
| --- | --- |
| Accelerometer | Measures the acceleration |
| Barometer | Sensor that can measure atmospheric pressure. |
| Magnetometer | It is able to detect magnetic fields |
| Gyroscope | Sensor that can provide orientation information. |
| Proximity sensor | This sensor lets the system know that you're most probably in a call and that the screen has to be turned off |
| Environment sensors | Moisture, humidity and temperature measurements |
| Thermometer | for measuring temperature |
| Air humidity sensor | for measuring air humidity |
| Pedometer | sensor used for counting the number of steps that the user has taken |
| Heart rate sensor | it is made to measure one's pulse |
| Fingerprint sensor | For Security |
| Hall Sensor | recognizes whether the cover is open or closed |
| RGB Light Sensor | measures the intensity of the light |
| Gesture Sensor | recognizes hand movements by detecting infrared rays that are reflected from the user's palm |
| Infrared Sensors | Distance & Range measurements |
| Force Sensors | Determines the pressure |
| Localization (GPS) Sensors | Location finding |
| Cameras | Capture the picture |

Typical functions of Smart Phones are as follows: Mobile browser, E-mail, Messaging, video calling, speakerphone, GPS, Stills and video camera functions, photo and video viewing and editing, E-book reading, apps (games, education, and utilities), media player, etc.

The smart phones make use of many wireless communication techniques like GSM, WIFI, Bluetooth, Zigbee, etc. These techniques allow mobile phones to be more useful for healthcare applications. Bluetooth is a technology for wireless communication. It is designed to replace cable connections. It connects small devices like mobile phones, PDAs and TVs using a short-range wireless connection. And it uses the 2.45 GHz frequency band. The connection can be point-to-point or multipoint where the maximum range is 10 meters. The transfer rate of the data is 1Mbps (or a maximum of 2Mbps).

*Table 2. Components of Mobile phone*

| I/O Devices | Processor or Microcontroller | Operating Systems / Software Modules |
|---|---|---|
| Key switches, LED, LCD, Buzzer, Camera, Sensors, Accelerometer Barometer Magnetometer Gyroscope Proximity sensor Environment sensors Thermometer Air humidity sensor Pedometer Heart rate sensor Fingerprint sensor Hall Sensor RGB Light Sensor Gesture Sensor Infrared Sensors<br><br>Force Sensors Localization (GPS) Sensors | 8051 PIC ARM AVR | Symbian Windows Palm OS iOS Android Bada |

# Hardware and Software Requirements

The following are the hardware and software requirements to develop the embedded system namely cell phone:

1.  Microcontroller or Microprocessor
2.  Accelerometer and other sensors
3.  LEDs / 7-Segment LEDS
4.  LCD
5.  Key Switches or Buttons
6.  Buzzer or Speaker
7.  ADC /DAC
8.  GSM / GPRS Modem
9.  Mobile Phone
10. SIM Card
11. Power supply / Battery
12. Connecting Wires / PCB
13. IDE Environment for writing program and testing and debugging
14. EPROM Program Downloader and Other necessary components and tools

## Mobile Operating Systems

- **Symbian:** Symbian is a mobile operating system designed for smartphones originally developed by Symbian Ltd. but currently maintained by Accenture.
- **Windows:** Microsoft Windows CE and abbreviated as WinCE is an operating system developed by Microsoft forEmbedded systems.
- **Palm OS:** Palm OS (also known as Garnet OS) is a mobile operating system initially developed by Palm, Inc., for personalDigital Assistants (PDAs) in 1996. Palm OS is designed for ease of use with a touchscreen-based graphical userInterface.
- **iOS:** iOS (previously iPhone OS) is a mobile operating system developed and distributed by Apple Inc. Originally released in 2007 for the iPhone and iPod Touch, it has been extended to support other Apple devices such as the iPad and Apple TV.
- **Android:** Android is a Linux-based operating system designed primarily for touchscreen mobile devices such as smartphones and tablet computers, developed by Google in conjunction with the Open Handset Alliance
- **Bada:** Bada is an operating system for mobile devices such as smartphones and tablet computers. It is developed by Samsung Electronics. Its name is derived from bada, meaning "ocean" or "sea" in Korean. It ranges from mid-range to high-end smartphones

## The Future of Surgery: Robotics a Case Study

Now days the robots are involved for the hospital assistant device. They do more work as a doctor. They are the examples for embedded system. The Tamil movie Enthiran has demonstrated how the robots are helpful for surgery (see Figure 2).

The following are few requirements to achieve the above robots for hospital management.

- Database design
- Form design for user controls
- Hardware integration
- Software coding, testing and debugging
- Simulation and prototyping

*Figure 2. Robotics in Surgery*

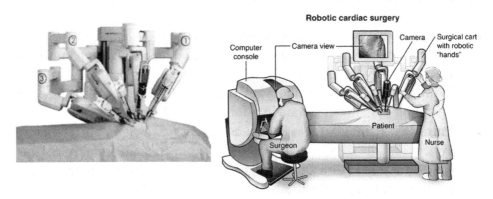

Exercise questions:

1. What is an embedded system? Draw the basic blocks of an embedded system?
2. What is mobile computing? How it is useful to health domain?
3. List any 15 sensors used for patient monitoring applications?
4. Discuss the various features of smart phone?
5. Draw the schematic diagram and write a simulation program to blink an LED when key switch is pressed?
6. Identify and list any 10 mobile APP's meant for future Health care domain?
7. What is Bluetooth? Write short notes on Bluetooth?
8. Illustrate how the data transfer takes place from device to device using wireless communication methods with an example?
9. Draw the block diagram patient care system?
10. Discuss the various wireless communication systems?

# REFERENCES

Kay, M., Santos, J., & Takane, M. (2011). mHealth: New horizons for health through mobile technologies. *World Health Organization, 64*(7), 66-71.

Manjula. (n.d.). *Lab manual on mobile application development lab.* Dept of Information Technology, Institute of Aeronautical Engineering Dundigal.

Moorthi, M. N., & Vaideeswaran, J. (n.d.). *Design of an Embedded System for Health Monitoring and Emergency services using wearable sensors.* Academic Press.

Narayana Moorthi & Manjula. (n.d.). Developing a framework for automated patient care monitoring system for medical clinics using 8051 microcontroller. *IJPBS*.

Nosrati, M., Karimi, R., & Hasanvand, H. A. (2012). Mobile computing: Principles, devices and operating systems. *World Applied Programming*, 2(7), 399–408.

Ozkil, A. G., Fan, Z., Dawids, S., Aanes, H., Kristensen, J. K., & Christensen, K. H. (2009, August). Service robots for hospitals: A case study of transportation tasks in a hospital. In *Automation and Logistics, 2009. ICAL'09. IEEE International Conference on* (pp. 289-294). IEEE. 10.1109/ICAL.2009.5262912

Rajan, Spanias, Ranganath, Banavar, & Spanias. (n.d.). *Health Monitoring Laboratories by Interfacing Physiological Sensors to Mobile Android Devices.* SenSIPCenter, School of ECEE, Arizona State University.

Stankevich, E., Paramonov, I., & Timofeev, I. (2012, April). Mobile phone sensors in health applications. In *Proc. 12th Conf. of Open Innovations Association FRUCT and Seminar on e-Tourism* (pp. 136-141). Academic Press.

# Chapter 5
# Mobile Patient Surveillance

**H. Parveen Sultana**
*VIT University, India*

**Nalini Nagendran**
*VIT University, India*

## ABSTRACT

*Surveillance is defined as providing security in critical situations or monitoring certain places where safety and security are important. Surveillance takes the lead in healthcare departments or sections. Surveillance is also helpful in diagnosing the errors that occur in the automated systems and happening of adverse events in patient care. The main objective of patient surveillance is to observe the changes that occur in any patient's health to provide appropriate medication through automation process. Initially, the comparison is made between surveillance and monitoring. Later the chapter discusses the wireless technologies and mobile applications used for patient surveillance. Using mobile healthcare systems surveillance data that includes not only patient's clinical information but also analyses clinical scenario periodically, the clinical information gathered is disseminated among various teams of specialists for decision making. The advancement in wireless devices not only monitors the patient's conditions but also provides required information or data. This is possible only when sensed data is communicated at an appropriate time to avoid unexpected events in critical care units. This wireless technology helps the nursing staff in improving the surveillance and guaranteeing patient's safety. This chapter explores mobile patient surveillance.*

DOI: 10.4018/978-1-5225-5036-5.ch005

# INTRODUCTION

In recent years, Surveillance (Makary&Daniel,2016) (Henneman, Gawlinski, & Giuliano,2012). play important role in patient observation. This process is executed by Health Care Professionals (HCP) (Mickan, Tilson, Atherton, Roberts, & Heneghan, 2013). to protect patients from inevitable and unavoidable situations that occur in acute and critical care sections. Surveillance has three functions such as data collection, clinical decision making, investigation and interpretation of data. There are more chances of medical error (Makary & Daniel, 2016) (Henneman, Gawlinski, & Giuliano, 2012) and adverse event (Henneman, Gawlinski, & Giuliano, 2012) occurrences with the hospitalized patients. Because each patient has more data that need to be processed by consultants based on their clinical decisions.

Medical errors are the main cause of patient disability, prolong hospital stay and even it may lead to demise. Institute of Medicine (IOM) (Kohn, Corrigan,& Donaldson, 2000) submitted a report on estimated death rate associated with medical errors (Makary & Daniel, 2016) in the USA and has concluded that 44,000 to 98,000 deaths occur annually. In 2013 the death rate estimated in the USA was around 2, 51,454 (James, 2013), due to medical errors. Medical errors are identified as the third leading cause of death in the USA (Makary & Daniel, 2016). The possible situations medical error occurs while diagnosing the disease when prescribing medicines without cognizance, device fault and lack of communication between physicians about the patient.

Adverse events (Henneman, Gawlinski, & Giuliano, 2012) are associated with medical errors. This is possible due to less attention towards the patient like the physician is not giving appropriate medication and patient is not acquiring proper quantity at right time. Adverse events are preventable because they can be avoidable with proper medical care and prevention program. Adverse events may not be avoidable in some situations, for example, unknown allergy reaction to a patient who is taking particular medicine for first time prescribed by the physician. Otherwise, it is preventable if prior information about the medicine is known to the physician. Figure 1 depicts the relationship between medical error and the adverse event. Generally the medical errors can be prevented but still few adverse events are unavoidable. The main cause for medical errors and adverse events are human negligence and device fault.

*Figure 1. Relationship between Medical Error and Adverse Event*

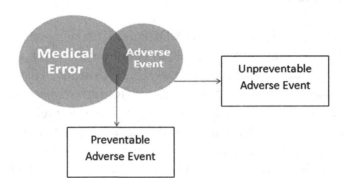

There are other medical errors and adverse events occur during medical treatment in hospitals. In order to provide a solution to this problem, many approaches need to be automated under the supervision of medical experts. Mobile devices and healthcare applications are widely used to automate the above-said approaches.

Preventing and identifying medical errors in the early stage of patient monitoring (Makary & Daniel, 2016) (Henneman, Gawlinski, & Giuliano, 2012) is used to detect life-threatening complications and to improve the safety of patients. Monitoring is a continuous process which is part of surveillance also. Since it is continual, the status of critical care patient disease alert the caregivers to save patients from life-threatening events. The data collected from the patient observation is based on resource availability and risk of assessment. The following Table 1 lists the difference between surveillance and monitoring.

*Table 1. Difference between Surveillance and Monitor*

| Surveillance | Monitoring |
|---|---|
| **Active Process** | **Passive Process** |
| Early Identification of medical risk and provide attention to the critical care patients. And attempt to prevent the medical error and adverse events. | Routine observation of a patient. It is part of surveillance and more specific. |
| Continuously analyze the patient's data which makes the clinical decision process easy. | It only records the medical data from the patient. |
| The physician may understand the changes occur in a patient during treatment which is usual or not. | It may not know the difference between patient's condition which is common or not. |
| It plays important role in saving the patient from life-threating events. | It records the patient's condition based on available resources and assessment procedures. |

It has been noticed that in most of the hospitals when amendment occurs in the structural organization, it affects the patient. As a result of this change, most of the care processes get altered and lead to a happening of adverse events. To overcome the above-said issues, nurse care is most important in the critical sections of hospitals. Caregivers should be aware as well as trained to notice the changes that occur in the system beforehand. This is to avoid hindrance in the investigation and special care of bedside patients by the caregivers. To accomplish the assigned task or job effectively, caregivers have to associate with the consultants and practiced to handle the unavoidable situations.

# BACKGROUND

## Patient Surveillance Through Mobile Devices and Applications

Patient Surveillance through a mobile device and its applications (apps) provide more flexibility in communication between HCPs and patient. This is known as Mobile Healthcare (mhealthcare) system. There are a variety of services provided by mobile apps wirelessly like prescribing medicines, vaccination and medical alerts, physician/hospital locators, appointment schedule, diagnose and treatment remotely.

HCPs can monitor patient's health condition remotely through mobile device and apps. Mobile device and apps collect information from patients apart and send it to the server for storing in the medical database. Then, HCPs analyses the information with the existing record of the patient and provide an appropriate solution to them. HCPs use healthcare to monitor patient's health and communicate with another physician in different locations via a mobile device.

Benefits of mobile device and apps (Mickan, Tilson, Atherton, Roberts, & Heneghan, 2013; Aungst, 2013) used by the patient are listed below:

- **Minimizing the Cost:** Monitoring patients in real time which avoid physician's regular visits.
- **Real-Time Disease Supervision:** Remote monitoring of patients treated actively before their condition worsens.

- **Enhanced Quality of Life:** Though patients are situated in various places, their medical conditions are monitored via a mobile device.
- **Enriched User Experience:** Patients can directly communicate with the medical professionals to clarify their suspicions.

All the leading companies like Microsoft, Apple, and Google are marketing their products and apps for healthcare. PatientKeeper (Mosa, Yoo, & Sheets, 2012) and Teamviewer (O'Neill, Holmer, Greenberg, & Meara, 2013) are apps that can be accessed by patient and physician via Apple and Android mobile devices. It can access remote data which is stored in desktop PCs also. X-Rays and image scans also can be viewed using Mobile MIM (O'Neill, Holmer, Greenberg, & Meara, 2013) open source Apple (O'Neill, Holmer, Greenberg, & Meara, 2013) apps available in the market. The patient monitoring system has developed to monitor Incentive Care Unit (ICU) (Mosa, Yoo, & Sheets, 2012) patients which produce alarm based patient's status. Rehabilitation centers also use mobile devices efficiently to monitor patient's activities. MobiSante (Ozdalga, Ozdalga, A.& Ahuja, 2012) was the first company to use mobile based diagnostic tool to take ultrasound investigation for Electrocardiogram (ECG) (Ren, Werner, Pazzi,& Boukerche, 2010) authorized by Food and Drug Administration (FDA) in 2011.

## Importance of Mobile Device and Apps

Mobile devices play a vital role in monitoring acute and critical care patient's health remotely. Mobile device apps are used to collect patient's data. Therefore HCPs analyze and interpret data to choose clinical decision processes in treating the patients effortlessly. HCPs mainly use mobile devices and apps for administration, patient record maintenance, communication, and consultation, etc. Patient's life becomes more secure by using mobile devices and apps. Some important tasks are listed below (Mickan, Tilson, Atherton, Roberts, & Heneghan, 2013; Aungst, 2013):

- Send periodic educational information and motivational guidance to drug addicts or chain-smokers who are trying to quit.
- Use Global Positioning System (GPS) to locate asthmatics to alert about weather conditions that may cause asthma attacks.
- Motivate the patients to do exercises through mobile apps.

- Alert diabetic patients about calorie consumption (food) based on their glucose and cholesterol level.
- Send medicine reminders and dosage intake to elderly patients at home.
- Track patient's location who is suffering from Alzheimer's disease using mobile GPS.
- The disabled persons can live their life independently with the help of smart devices.

## Research Areas in Mobile Healthcare

Mobile devices and apps are used immensely inpatient surveillance. Still, there are few areas to be identified and need improvement as mentioned by World Health Organization (WHO) (Kay, Santos, &Takane, 2011). WHO has identified fourteen categories of mobile health services which are helpful in improving Quality of Service (QoS) (Kay, Santos, & Takane, 2011):

- **Telephone Help Lines for Healthcare:** Healthcare professionals deliver advice about health through portable devices to the people.
- **Free Telephone Services for Medical Emergency:** This service is used to connect health care professionals directly and acquire their assistance during a medical emergency.
- **Emergencies and Disaster Management:** Mobile services are highly desired in natural disaster and emergency situations because wired network communication is not feasible.
- **Mobile Telemedicine:** Short Messaging Service (SMS) widely used by chronic disease patient at home to communicate with HCPs.
- **Reminders About Appointment:** Voice or SMS services used to remind the patient's appointments and infant's immunization schedule.
- **Community Mobilization and Health Preferment:** Mostly government send SMS alerts about vaccination schedule to gestation women or parents (for infants) and encourage people to care about their health.
- **Treatment Compliance:** This service is used to support chronic disease patients by sending voice and SM. The main goal is to improve treatment compliance, disease eradication and overcoming challenges such as drug resistance.

- **Mobile Patient Records:** Information about patients is stored in the form of Electronic Medical Record (EMR) through mobile technologies. So the record can be accessed anytime from anywhere.
- **Information Access:** Many healthcare databases provide access to data at any point of time.
- **Monitoring Patients:** Monitor and treat the patient's illness distantly.
- **Health Surveys and Data Collection:** Conduct health surveys through mobile devices and alert them accordingly.
- **Surveillance:** Disease surveillance through mobile technologies used for collecting patient information and tracks their health conditions.
- **Raising Awareness About Health:** Conduct social programs to educate people on health care.
- **Decision Support Systems:** Software programs are used to help HCPs on clinical decision-making process with help of patient's medical history.

The above-mentioned services are expected to be developed more. In future, mobile device storage needs to be increased because patient and HCPs want to store voluminous data. The patient self-monitoring and prevention of diseases are important than all, so apps are expected to fulfill process of patient monitoring.

## Wireless Technologies in Patient Monitoring

Recently there are various wireless technologies used in mobile healthcare systems. These technologies are a part of patient observation which provides effective mechanisms for patient surveillance. In most of the hospitals, mobile healthcare (healthcare) (Ren,Werner,Pazzi,& Boukerche, 2010) had shown a vigorous growth in the patient monitoring and helpful for the healthcare organizations through policy agents. Mobile healthcare system challenges to deliver healthcare amenities to critical and emergency patients all the seven days twenty-four hours determinedly. This is only possible when wireless devices connected with the mobile healthcare systems. These wireless devices may be of wearable or deployable types that are coupled with the mobile healthcare systems for communication wirelessly. This type of connectivity improves the effectiveness of the telemedicine (Ren,Werner, Pazzi,& Boukerche, 2010) systems. A major concern in the mobile healthcare system is to maintain the confidentiality of patient's information by providing secured communication.

Mobile healthcare systems enhanced to the level of electronic healthcare (healthcare) (Ren,Werner,Pazzi,& Boukerche, 2010) which provides services in real time. A healthcare is accessible by professionals in hospitals and medical institutions to monitor the patients remotely or at specified intervals. Patients get benefited from ehealthcare by getting suggestions and medicines from mhealthcare and telemedicine systems. Wireless technologies have a good impact in mhealthcare in achieving its goals practically or realistically. Most of the nursing centers that are connected wirelessly take guidance and receive medical advice from the associated hospitals or medical institutions. The involvement of wireless technology such as mobile and wearable devices had made the healthcare system healthier in terms of medical. These manageable and wearable devices are the backbone of mhealthcare systems by sensing and gathering patient's data frequently to disseminate to the nursing centers or healthcare systems.

## Architecture of mhealthcare System

Mobile healthcare systems get benefitted from the wireless technologies like Mobile Ad Hoc Networks (MANETs) (Ren,Werner,Pazzi,& Boukerche, 2010) and Body Sensor Networks (BSNs) (Ren,Werner,Pazzi,& Boukerche, 2010). These networks are helpful in well organized and distributed healthcare systems with an appropriate wireless infrastructure. Because of this wireless structure, more patients will have maximum opportunity to get treatment timely inside the hospitals or remote healthcare centers. This is to avoid last minute emergency by providing the first level of medical care. Since the healthcare structure is wirelessly connected most of the procedures (to be executed) are dependent on wireless medical devices. These devices transmit the sensed and gathered data to the relevant sections in a secure and reliable way.

The architecture of mobile healthcare system is depicted in Figure 2. The mhealthcare system has various monitoring devices which are connected with the internet server which is called as response server (Ren,Werner,Pazzi,& Boukerche, 2010). In this architecture, it has been shown that medical professionals and the medical transports always get connected with the center server for providing appropriate services at right time. There is more possibility that medical information is hacked by unwanted invaders while the information is transmitted between the medical centers. Mobile healthcare system should

*Figure 2. mhealthcare System Architecture*

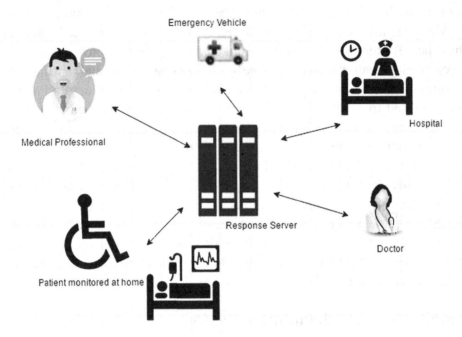

maintain some security mechanisms in the communication process to avoid the intervention of unauthorized access. Since mobile healthcare system is a collection of wireless medical devices, it is necessary that more security is provided in the dynamic and widespread health environments.

Wireless technologies are used in various medical places such as telemedicine system, monitoring assisted living people in the home, exchange of medical information and robotic surgery. The mobile healthcare system is very much needed in rural places where the facilities have to be provided through mobile communication. Mobile healthcare system had helped the professionals and other medical specialists to handle the inaccessible situations without any pre-structure requirement. Mobile communication has created a revolution in the day to day lives of people in the medical field. This is only possible through wireless technologies like IEEE 802.11, IEEE 802.15.4, Bluetooth and WiFi (Ren,Werner,Pazzi,& Boukerche, 2010). These wireless technologies help the medical professionals and doctors to access patient's information round-the-clock. In mhealthcare system sensors play a major role in observing the patient's conditions.

Most of the well-developed countries use the mhealthcare system for observing the activities of elderly people in houses or those who require assistance with medical devices. As Body sensor network is a part of the mhealthcare system, it is helpful in predicting the medical conditions of patients earlier. The sensors involved in the BSN observe patient's condition, gather data and transmit to the medical centers for further actions. BSN with mhealthcare system remind about the medicines or tests to be conducted through frequent or timely messages. Because of this computerized process, most of the administrative costs are reduced. In other words the sensor devices act as Personal Digital Assistants (PDAs) (Ren,Werner,Pazzi,& Boukerche, 2010) to maintain patient's health records such as level of blood pressure, blood glucose level, Electroencephalogram (EEG) (Ren,Werner,Pazzi,& Boukerche, 2010), Electromyogram (EMG) (Ren,Werner,Pazzi,& Boukerche, 2010) and ECG. This reduces the risk of patient falling sick which lead to unpredicted situations.

## Mobile Healthcare System With Sensor Devices

Following are few difficulties in a mhealthcare system that require more attention during data exchange in real time.

- Consistency in patient nursing
- Durability of medical devices
- Perspective of patient information
- Safety and security of medical data

All the above-said issues can be resolved through MANET, provided the wireless structure should have safe, consistent and effective necessities in data transmission. The wearable sensor devices in BSN have fast data rate with short transmission capability. As sensors collect patient's data it consumes energy so at regular intervals the batteries of wearable devices to be changed. The wireless structure associated with the mhealthcare system is centralized and distributed manner to share its characteristics. Whenever a patient with wearable devices wanders from one place to another place, the topology of wireless structure also changes. Amendments in the wireless structure coordinate with the mhealthcare system to fetch patient's data at an appropriate time. The portability of patient creates adaptability in the mhealthcare system for the smooth transmission of patient data.

Wearable devices observe both inpatients and outpatients medical conditions. These devices send two types of indications to the medical centers. They are routine messages (Ren,Werner,Pazzi,& Boukerche, 2010) and emergency messages (Ren,Werner,Pazzi,& Boukerche, 2010). Routine messages usually hold periodic information about patient's vibrant conditions. Emergency messages send information about patient's critical conditions for which preference to be given first. The sensor devices are deployed in such a way that emergency data is transmitted with the highest priority. Various methods have been applied to reduce the consumption of energy during transmission by the wearable devices. In the mhealthcare system, energy consumption is the main factor while handling critical scenarios of emergency situations.

## Body Sensor Networks (BSN)

A wireless structure comprised of small, low-cost, wearable or deployable sensors are called Body Area Network (BAN) (Ren,Werner,Pazzi,& Boukerche, 2010). It is also referred as Body Sensor Network (BSN) (Ren,Werner,Pazzi,& Boukerche, 2010). In BAN life of the wearable sensor is dependable on its battery utilization. Timely replacement of batteries in wearable sensors helps to maintain collection and dissemination of patient data at a required time. These sensor devices use Bluetooth, IEEE 802.11, IEEE 802.15.4 and General Packet Radio Service (GPRS) (Ren,Werner,Pazzi,& Boukerche, 2010) as wireless technologies for data transmission. BSN connect medical devices with sensors directly for timely information. The topology of Body Sensor Network is shown in Figure 3.

BSN is also called as Wireless BAN (WBAN) (Ren, Werner, Pazzi, & Boukerche, 2010) which comprised of computing wearable devices. The portable devices can be used in any fabric pockets, attached on any surface of the human body or implanted inside the body. These devices are monitored through wireless devices like mobile phones, medical sensors, and smart devices. Smart devices are used in Wireless Personal Area Networks (WPANs) (Boukerche &Ren, 2009) to improve the performance of patient monitoring. WPAN is helpful in diagnosing patient's conditions or critical signs that occur in and around patient's body. The smart (sensor) devices involved in WPAN are mostly connected with the internet. So, if any emergency or medical assistance is required immediately care or medication should be provided.

*Figure 3. Topology of BSN*

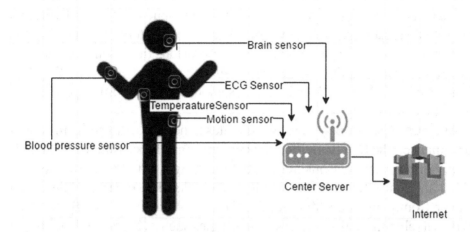

Actually, WBAN and WPAN use Zigbee (Ren, Werner, Pazzi, & Boukerche, 2010) wireless technology as an important factor in data communication. This smart network is the next level of the mhealthcare system which connects various fields like medical, engineering and automated computation. This combination is called as Wearable and Implantable BSN (WIBSN) (Darwish & Hassanien, 2011). The layout of WIBSN is shown in Figure 4.

*Figure 4. Overview of WIBSN*

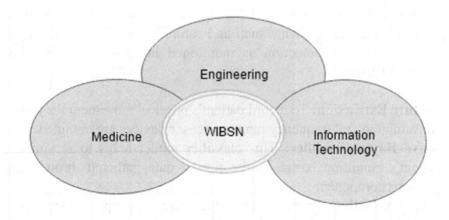

In the recent year's research had been focused on new developments in wireless sensor medical devices. Enhancement in the Micro-Electro-Mechanical Systems (MEMS) (Darwish & Hassanien, 2011) and wireless transmissions had raised the level of mhealthcare systems. Because of this new improvement the sensor devices used in various fields sense, gather and actuate according to the conditions set in it. The involvement of Wireless Sensor Network (WSN) (Darwish & Hassanien, 2011) gives a new perspective to the mhealthcare system.

As a part of WSN, BAN has two modules in healthcare to perform patient surveillance. The first module called Personal Data Processing Unit (PDPU) (Ren,Werner,Pazzi,& Boukerche, 2010) manages all the sensor devices which are connected with the wireless networks. The other module called Sensor Communication Module (SCM) (Ren,Werner,Pazzi,& Boukerche, 2010) which utilizes the wireless technologies such as Zigbee or WiFi to get connected with PDPU. Considering patient's psychological and physiological factor neural network concept is added to analyze the patient's condition. Moreover many Artificial Intelligence (AI) (Ren,Werner,Pazzi,& Boukerche, 2010) techniques applied in mhealthcare monitoring. These AI techniques help the medical professionals to observe patient's ailments which are caused by variations in body temperature or the environment. The involvement of AI in BSN is to reduce the risk of fetching irrelevant information gathered by the medical sensors.

The method applied in BSN to diagnose patient's medical ailment is Incremental Diagnosis Method (IDM) (Ren,Werner,Pazzi,& Boukerche, 2010). This methodology senses patient's illness through the wearable sensor devices. These medical devices record the vigorous change of sensed data according to patient's conditions. IDM is an AI based reasoning procedure comprised of three components such as Feature Extraction, Naïve Bayes Classifier and Sensor Selection as mentioned in (Ren,Werner,Pazzi,& Boukerche, 2010):

- **Feature Extraction:** To record patient's physical movement the power consumption and frequency range of sensor devices are obtained.
- **Naïve Bayes Classifier:** This classifier model helps to reckon the patient's condition based on the sensed data gathered through the previous component
- **Sensor Selection:** On reception of the sensed data appropriate action or medication to be decided which improves the state of patients.

Though wireless technology is a part of the mhealthcare system in patient monitoring, initially it requires few sensor devices to diagnose the state of patients. To perform appropriate tasks like medication, emergency treatment mhealthcare system requires additional sensors to monitor patients' conditions vigorously. This is only possible through BSN, WPAN, and WIBAN. With the help of these wireless technologies, patients can be monitored continuously by observing vital conditions such as symptoms of heart attack, declination of insulin levels and fluctuation of blood pressure. Moreover, the mhealthcare system is involved in the fields of military, security, and sports to provide seamless communication between professionals (persons) or professionals (individuals) and machines.

## Reliable and Secured Patient Monitoring

Security and privacy are two important factors in the mhealthcare system. Since most of the medical, as well as confidential data, are exchanged between the center servers and end users, importance should be given in securing these data. Consistent and secure software used to provide authentication during data transmission since in wireless communication data is vulnerable to attackers. So an effective secure mhealthcare system should be implemented to handle remote monitoring of patients secured way.

## Reliable Patient Monitoring

Consistent and dependable, continuous network access is essential in wireless patient health monitoring. This is accomplished by utilizing various wireless structures available in the specified location. The changes occur in patient's health to be carried by several data packets and combined as a whole before transmitting to the medical professionals or HCPs. This reliable wireless structure able to monitor and provide medical information under following situations as mentioned in (Varshney, 2007):

- **Network Breakdown:** When network disconnected or malfunction in devices, the medical information to be obtained from the local network.
- **Restricted Access:** Due to interference or improper transmissions, patients should be monitored through temporary resources.

- **Interrupted Connectivity:** During natural calamities or some mishaps caregivers able to connect with the patients through wired communication.

The response server of the dependable wireless network should have the capability to connect with the other reliable network under the above-said scenarios. The interchange of the wireless network is possible only if the medical devices of smart sensor devices type to realize the change of network connectivity. Also, have the portability and adaptability to fit in any type of wireless network to resume its monitoring processes. The interchange of network access depends upon the bandwidth capacity, data transmission range and power consumption level of sensor nodes involved in it. To overcome the issues of network exchange in the healthcare system, a strong multi-network architecture access with smart resources should be formed. But the recent wireless technology (4G) allows users to toggle between various wireless technologies.

In a dependable wireless network, health monitoring with reliable data delivery is most important. The constant monitoring of patients and recording their vital conditions are quite difficult in the healthcare system. Inconsistency and unstable quality of network could result in interrupting constant patient observation and dissemination of medical data to the HCPs. Due to delayed responses, patient's condition gets worse. To enhance consistency of wireless health monitoring structure the following developments are required:

- Broadcast or multicast transmission to be applied.
- Automatic power cut-off mechanism in sensor devices.
- Effective end-to-end reliability (Varshney, 2007) using integrated protocol standard.

## Security Approach in Patient Observation

As wireless technologies provide effective connectivity between response servers and professionals, a concern is how securely medical data is exchanged. In the mhealthcare system, there are possibilities that confidential or medical information can be hacked by the intruders. Since mhealthcare system comprised of combined resources, mobile handlers and wireless connectivity, the complexity of security level also increases. To overcome this issue many security based methodologies such as encryption and decryption technologies, session or private key generation have been applied during medical data exchange. The key generation is maintained at the response server and disseminated to the users who have been authenticated and registered in the mhealthcare system. To hold the confidentiality of medical data Elliptic-Curve Cryptography (ECC) (Ren,Werner,Pazzi,& Boukerche, 2010) is applied in the mhealthcare system. ECC reduce the task of public key generation and provide more security for user verification, digital signature (Ren,Werner,Pazzi,& Boukerche, 2010) and encoding process in professionals' and nursing users' mobiles. The following diagram (Figure 5) depicts the flow of security mechanism applied to patient's data.

According to Health Insurance Portability Accountability Act (HIPAA) (Ren,Werner,Pazzi,& Boukerche, 2010) regulations, the mhealthcare system provides security and privacy solutions. In the first level of the security process, each patient's details are registered in the response server along with the signed agreement. In the privacy process, each patient's information is encrypted and decrypted through the biometric smart card method. These two processes help the medical professionals and end users (authorized) to protect patients' information confidentially.

*Figure 5. Flow of security mechanism in Patient's data*

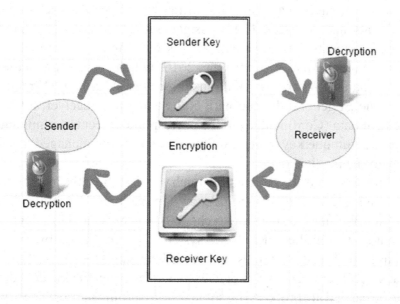

As explained in (Chakravorty, 2006) a health-related architecture called MobiCare (Chakravorty, 2006) that promises to offer patient monitoring with the secured transmission in various wireless scenarios. MobiCare is mainly meant for mobile patient care (Chakravorty, 2006). This architecture is configured in such a way that the medical sensor devices can be deployed, organized and triggered remotely. It also uses a software which has portability and compatibility with medical devices. The bidirectional transmission of diagnosed patient's information is executed through the internet servers connected to it. MobiCare had challenged to deliver patient care with less cost, which set a path to the next level of the mobile healthcare system.

## Key Mechanism in Patient Monitoring

A security key generation method is based on Electrocardiogram (EKG) (Ren,Werner,Pazzi,& Boukerche, 2010) signals. EKG signals based key method produces cryptographic keys (Ren,Werner,Pazzi,& Boukerche, 2010). The EKG key is produced from the EKG signals of the patients. In this approach, the generated key values vary from patient to patient, unlike traditional key mechanism. When two sensors in the BSN transmit to each other, it follows the procedure of EKG key generation for security purpose. The observed EKG signals are converted into binary data to create a common key before transmission. Since these sensors are in the region of BSN the common key is safely shared among the authorized peoples such as medical professionals and end users. The key is generated based on pulses produced from the heartbeats of the patient. This is recognized as Entity Identifier (EI) (Ren,Werner,Pazzi,& Boukerche, 2010) which is the main factor value in data exchange. Whenever data transmission is initiated BSN request for EI, once the EI get coordinated with both sender and receiver, it transmits the medical data (Confidential) to the corresponding center or nursing care section. This unique key generation method somehow managed to provide security to the medical data.

In addition to security, patients are much worried about the maintenance of their personal medical information. A new approach called Quality of Privacy (QoP) (Ren,Werner,Pazzi,& Boukerche, 2010) is presented to safeguard the confidential data in the mhealthcare system. The QoP is set by the patient or end user to observe activities that occur in around the wireless structure. Basically, QoP services such as data exchange between the medical devices, tasks to be carried are proposed by some self-governing parties. These parties do agree with the patient's QoP level which indicates the range of information to be shared. If the self-governing party does not meet the requirement of the QoP level then the privacy services will be assigned to some other agents.

## Smartphone Significance in the Healthcare System

Smartphones have changed the way of living and by using GPS smartphones get connected with the mhealthcare system. Smartphone takes a lead in providing health-related information through some application software which is installed in it. It has become a mediator for offering continuous service in the mhealthcare system. In healthcare fields, the smartphone is used as diagnosing device in the home, as an information provider in rural centers and as a supporter in disease treatment. Smartphones are very often used in rural places to monitor patient's conditions to offer appropriate treatment. Treatment is possible through the medical records that have been stored in those devices. Moreover, the elderly people with various disabilities who require personal assistance in medical care (medication) are given through the smartphones. The portability and compatibility feature of smartphone helps the mhealthcare system in gathering medical data and monitoring communal health centers. Smartphone also used in telemedicine and provide healthcare awareness remotely. It shows that smartphones are used not only for text or multimedia communication but being part of mhealthcare monitoring.

## Significance of Security and Confidentiality in Healthcare Applications

Though health care system connected with the wireless technologies for efficient data exchange, it has to maintain a certain level of confidentiality which should not vulnerable to hackers. According to (Henneman, Gawlinski, & Giuliano, 2012) following necessities shows how privacy and security are important in WIBSN:

- **Data Secrecy:** In mhealthcare systems during medical data exchange more prevention to be handled to maintain the confidentiality. Though patient's data is accessible by authorized personnel, during data transmission security mechanisms should be applied. This is to avoid the intervention of intruders by breaching the patient's information.

- **Data Verification:** The sensed medical data from medical sensor devices are interchanged between the unit care staff and the response server. So in any healthcare applications, the medical data should be verified with the professionals (sender) and response server (receiver).
- **Robust User Verification:** A powerful authentication process (like a digital signature or biometric approval) to be applied in the transmission of patient's data. Since mhealthcare applications are communicating wirelessly, it is desirable to perform robust verification between the nursing care unit and caretakers or medical professionals.
- **Data Consistency:** Most of the medical devices are of sensors. Due to mechanical or electrical faults that occur in sensor devices, incorrect data would be delivered. Therefore it is mandatory that suitable integrity processes be executed at the receiver end to avoid adversary intrusions.
- **Supply of Security Key:** A unique key mechanism (based on physiological or psychological changes) used to verify the patient's medical data. Professionals may use effective key generation methodologies to protect the medical data from the vulnerable attacks.
- **Managing Retrieval Process:** Users like caretakers, chemists, welfare people and insurance agents have direct access to patients or medical data. It is necessary that centralized process should be applied to limit the access of confidential and private data of patients.
- **Data Convenience:** In healthcare applications sensors round the clock operates in and around critical section patients. Moreover, sensors run on batteries, the power consumption of medical sensor devices to be checked and the information to be pooled in the centralized database at regular intervals. This is to ensure the availability of patient's medical conditions (data) to the nursing staff or medical professionals.
- **Data Originality:** However security and privacy take a lead in the mhealthcare system, précised data is most important. To avoid the false data distribution, patient's medical information to be collected and disseminated at discrete and stipulated intervals. Data retrieval may be of partial or complete shared type.
- **Secure GPS:** Healthcare applications can also be operated from rural regions. The patient's exact location should be identified through GPS tracker. This tracker tool helps mhealthcare system to secure medical data from unauthorized access globally.

- **Persistence of Medical Data:** Due to mechanical or battery failure, the medical sensor devices to be replaced. So when any replacement of sensor device is required, previous data to be stored and used as backup data for newly installed sensor devices.
- **Transmission and Estimation:** Most of the sensor devices are self-operated and remotely controlled. Medical sensor devices chosen for healthcare applications should achieve security and privacy processes cost effectively.
- **Patient Consent:** For research investigation, medical data is very much useful. Therefore, patient's medical history can be circulated by medical professionals for a discussion. This can be approved with a prior permission from patient's consent form.

Though healthcare applications utilize wireless technology, the wireless structure is vulnerable to cyber-attacks and experience device failures. So it is essential to maintain patient's previous and current medical diagnose reports in the cloud-based database for future recovery.

## Smart Patient Surveillance Application: A Case Study

Frequently patients at the age of sixties need substantially more care in terms of medication and physical activities due to inherently unavoidable weakness. In such times when the need arises, a common problem in the modern society is that people are unable to spend time with the old people whom it is essential.

Monitoring and medicine administration for the patients is a critical element as it is impossible to keep track of patients all the time. Also, the most problematic issues arise in the healthcare system which is due to medical errors. The drug underdose or overdose is due to erratic intake of medicine which is a concerning issue in patient's health. Silva et al. (2013) proposed SapoMed, which is a mobile health application for medical management. It manages and keeps track of all the prescribed medication to prevent the medical errors. This mobile app makes the users conscious about the medicine schedule by giving alert notification messages to them. Wang et al. (2009) proposed a patient medicine reminder system which takes the input of the drug prescription details of the patient and then displays the list of medicines that are to be taken by the patient at the suggested time.

Most of the systems mentioned above are related to medicine reminder and had some limitations like some of the applications were platform dependent as they were designed only for particular operating systems. Further SapoMed and WedJat (Silva, Lopes, Marques, Rodrigues, & Proença, 2013) applications were built for Android devices, not for the iPhone-based operating system (iOS). The existing systems did not synchronize medical reminders with multiple mobile devices. Also, there was no authentication mechanism to verify the identity of the user before adding some measures.

Hence to overcome these limitations, the proposed system designed web based Application, Android based Application, and iOS app to support multiple operating systems. This proposed application also uses Google OAuth (Boyd, 2012) to verify user identity.

The proposed system goals are shown in Figure 6 and have four components that are listed below:

- To provide medical care for the elderly patient and help them to consume medicines suggested by the practitioner at a specified time (Zao, Wang, Tsai, & Liu, 2010; Wang, Tsai, Liu, & Zao, 2009; Silva, Lopes, Marques, Rodrigues, & Proença, 2013).
- With help of this mobile app, they can control electrical appliances like fan, light and air conditioner.
- With the help of automated footlight control, elderly or physically challenged people can walk around the house at any time especially in the night.
- Smart walking stick (José, Farrajota, Rodrigues, & Du Buf, 2011; Loomis, Marston, Golledge, & Klatzky, 2005) helps the patients lot while walking and it gives the buzzer alarm when any obstacles occur in their path.

The proposed system has mainly four components. The first one is medicine reminder system which has two components such as software and hardware. Mobile app and web app are software which accepts user's input and then add reminders. Secondly, the hardware which uses Arduino (Niver, 2014) to select the box whose light is to be switched on at the time of medicine consumption and blowing the alarm to indicate the patient's medicine intake.

The second part of this system is home appliance control system which also has two parts: app and hardware interface with Arduino processor.

*Figure 6. Smart Patient Surveillance Applications*

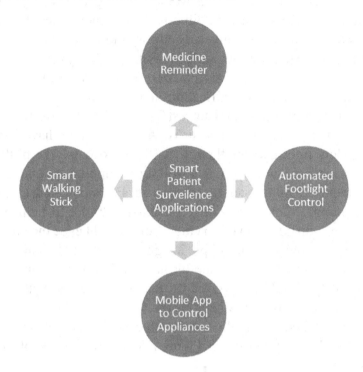

There are two apps web and mobile based. The web app is hosted on Heroku (Middleton & Schneeman, 2013) and the mobile app currently available for android devices. Its hardware interface includes Arduino processor which is connected to the appliances and it controls the operation of the devices.

The system's third part consists of automated footlight control system which controls the footlights and detects the nearby movements. If any movement occurs adjacently, the sensor will detect it and Arduino processor will enable the footlight. The last component of the system is Smart walking stick which detects the object in front of it. It informs the user (elder person or patient) about the obstacle (object) by blowing the buzzer and trigger the red LED or if the way is clear then the green LED glows.

These four smart surveillance applications provide a holistic solution to the elderly people who find trouble in daily activities. The objective of medicine reminder module is to remind the user about the medicine intake. The system is to make sure that the user never forgets to take the medicine and hence it reminds in three ways.

First, it has a visual indicator which would be the light. Secondly, it assumes that a person is not sitting close to pill box; he may not notice the lights. So it also has a buzzer which will give an auditory indication that the medicine needs to be taken. Suppose the patient is outside, the system has a mobile reminder app (Zao, Wang, Tsai, & Liu, 2010; Wang, Tsai, Liu, & Zao, 2009) which reminds using mobile notifications about the medication time.

The appliance control system is not just for the elderly to have a comfortable life, also about their safety and security. A lot of people have issues like visibility in low light and for them, it will be extremely helpful to have something reachable that helps in controlling the appliances and lights.

The obstacle detecting walking stick (José, Farrajota, Rodrigues, & Du Buf, 2011; Loomis, Marston, Golledge, & Klatzky, 2005) is to help the elderly people who have difficulty in observing (seeing) and hence they use a stick. So the idea is to provide some simple insights by giving red and green light indicators along with a buzzer for audible notification. This module also has a footlight that helps the elderly to go and access (drink water) anything at night or also to go to the restroom. Since it is dark at night and light switches are mostly away from beds, it's really comfortable for them if lights switched on automatically when they step down. Figure 7 depicts the process of automated footlight control system.

In future work, the proposed idea have been enhanced to add a database to the appliance control system which will keep a record of the user input for each appliance about the operation of an appliance like what time the user switches it on or switch off. So, then using that database the system can predict when the user will switch on which devices and when he will switch it off. Based on intelligence prediction approach, the system can control the devices in future in the automatic mode of the system.

In the medicine reminder system as a future work, it has been decided to add a confirmation from the user whether they have taken the medicine or not. If they haven't taken the medicine the information will be sent to the physician and he/she can reschedule the further medicine reminders according to the new schedule. Currently, the walking stick is only to detect front objects like wall, doors etc. In future, height and depth of objects are also considered in identifying hindrance about the stairs or any down step ahead. In the footlight, the new idea will be added as learning algorithm in future which would use the previous data to control the footlights before the user actually goes there.

*Figure 7. Automated Footlight Control System*

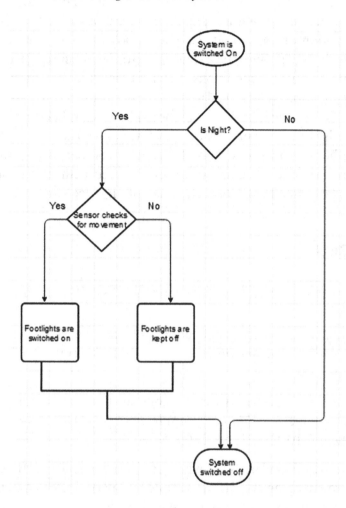

## CONCLUSION

Patient surveillance is to observe the changes that occur in any patient's health to provide appropriate medication through automation process. This chapter focuses on wireless technologies and mobile applications used for patient surveillance. Discussions were on how to prevent unpredictable events and provide solutions to have uninterrupted patient monitoring. It has been explained that mobile healthcare systems hold surveillance data which include not only patient's clinical information but also analyses clinical scenario periodically. The clinical information gathered to be disseminated among various teams of specialists for decision making. The advancement in wireless devices not only monitors the patient's conditions but also provides required information or data to HCPs. This is possible only when sensed data is communicated at an appropriate time to avoid unexpected errors (faults) that affect patient's conditions. Later a case study on smart patient surveillance application is elucidated to show the performance of assistance to elderly people. This application describes the applications related to medicine remainder, footlight movement control, smart walking stick and mobile app for controlling home appliances. This chapter ensures that today's world is more dependent on wireless technologies not only in the medical field but also in other fields like biomedical, Computational Intelligence and Engineering.

# REFERENCES

Adibi, S. (Ed.). (2015). *Mobile health: a technology road map* (Vol. 5). Springer.

Aungst, T. D. (2013). Medical applications for pharmacists using mobile devices. *The Annals of Pharmacotherapy, 47*(7-8), 1088–1095. doi:10.1345/aph.1S035 PMID:23821609

Boukerche, A., & Ren, Y. (2009). A secure mobile healthcare system using trust-based multicast scheme. *IEEE Journal on Selected Areas in Communications, 27*(4), 387–399. doi:10.1109/JSAC.2009.090504

Boulos, M. N. K., Wheeler, S., Tavares, C., & Jones, R. (2011). How smartphones are changing the face of mobile and participatory healthcare: An overview, with an example from eCAALYX. *Biomedical Engineering Online, 10*(1), 1. doi:10.1186/1475-925X-10-24 PMID:21466669

Boyd, R. (2012). *Getting started with OAuth 2.0.* O'Reilly Media, Inc.

Chakravorty, R. (2006). MobiCare: A programmable service architecture for mobile medical care. In *Fourth Annual IEEE International Conference on Pervasive Computing and Communications Workshops (PERCOMW'06)* (pp. 5). IEEE.

Darwish, A., & Hassanien, A. E. (2011). Wearable and implantable wireless sensor network solutions for healthcare monitoring. *Sensors (Basel), 11*(6), 5561–5595. doi:10.3390110605561 PMID:22163914

Henneman, E. A., Gawlinski, A., & Giuliano, K. K. (2012). Surveillance: A strategy for improving patient safety in acute and critical care units. *Critical Care Nurse, 32*(2), e9–e18. doi:10.4037/ccn2012166 PMID:22467622

James, J. T. (2013). A new, evidence-based estimate of patient harms associated with hospital care. *Journal of Patient Safety, 9*(3), 122–128. doi:10.1097/PTS.0b013e3182948a69 PMID:23860193

José, J., Farrajota, M., Rodrigues, J. M., & Du Buf, J. H. (2011). The SmartVision local navigation aid for blind and visually impaired persons. *International Journal of Digital Content Technology and its Applications, 5*(5), 362-375.

Kay, M., Santos, J., & Takane, M. (2011). mHealth: New horizons for health through mobile technologies. *World Health Organization, 64*(7), 66-71.

Kohn, L. T., Corrigan, J. M., & Donaldson, M. S. (Eds.). (2000). *To err is human: building a safer health system* (Vol. 6). National Academies Press.

Kumar, P., & Lee, H. J. (2011). Security issues in healthcare applications using wireless medical sensor networks: A survey. *Sensors (Basel), 12*(1), 55–91. doi:10.3390120100055 PMID:22368458

Loomis, J. M., Marston, J. R., Golledge, R. G., & Klatzky, R. L. (2005). Personal guidance system for people with visual impairment: A comparison of spatial displays for route guidance. *Journal of Visual Impairment & Blindness, 99*(4), 219. PMID:20054426

Makary, M. A., & Daniel, M. (2016). Medical error—the third leading cause of death in the US. *BMJ (Clinical Research Ed.), 353*, i2139. PMID:27143499

Mickan, S., Tilson, J. K., Atherton, H., Roberts, N. W., & Heneghan, C. (2013). Evidence of effectiveness of health care professionals using handheld computers: A scoping review of systematic reviews. *Journal of Medical Internet Research, 15*(10), 212. doi:10.2196/jmir.2530 PMID:24165786

Middleton, N., & Schneeman, R. (2013). *Heroku: Up and Running.* O'Reilly Media, Inc.

Mosa, A. S. M., Yoo, I., & Sheets, L. (2012). A systematic review of healthcare applications for smartphones. *BMC Medical Informatics and Decision Making, 12*(1), 1. doi:10.1186/1472-6947-12-67 PMID:22781312

Niver, H. M. (2014). *Getting to Know Arduino*. The Rosen Publishing Group.

O'Neill, K. M., Holmer, H., Greenberg, S. L., & Meara, J. G. (2013). Applying surgical apps: Smartphone and tablet apps prove useful in clinical practice. *Bulletin of the American College of Surgeons, 98*(11), 10–18. PMID:24313133

Ozdalga, E., Ozdalga, A., & Ahuja, N. (2012). The smartphone in medicine: A review of current and potential use among physicians and students. *Journal of Medical Internet Research, 14*(5), e128. doi:10.2196/jmir.1994 PMID:23017375

Ren, Y., Werner, R., Pazzi, N., & Boukerche, A. (2010). Monitoring patients via a secure and mobile healthcare system. *IEEE Wireless Communications, 17*(1), 59–65. doi:10.1109/MWC.2010.5416351

Silva, B. M., Lopes, I. M., Marques, M. B., Rodrigues, J. J., & Proença, M. L. (2013). A mobile health application for outpatient's medication management. In *2013 IEEE International Conference on Communications (ICC)* (pp. 4389-4393). IEEE. 10.1109/ICC.2013.6655256

Valentin, A., Capuzzo, M., Guidet, B., Moreno, R. P., Dolanski, L., Bauer, P., & Metnitz, P. G. (2006). Patient safety in intensive care: Results from the multinational Sentinel Events Evaluation (SEE) study. *Intensive Care Medicine, 32*(10), 1591–1598. doi:10.100700134-006-0290-7 PMID:16874492

Varshney, U. (2007). Pervasive healthcare and wireless health monitoring. *Mobile Networks and Applications, 12*(2-3), 113–127. doi:10.100711036-007-0017-1

Wang, M. Y., Tsai, P. H., Liu, J. W. S., & Zao, J. K. (2009). Wedjat: a mobile phone based medicine intake reminder and monitor. In *Bioinformatics and BioEngineering, 2009. BIBE'09. Ninth IEEE International Conference on.* (pp. 423-430). IEEE.

Zao, J. K., Wang, M. Y., Tsai, P., & Liu, J. W. (2010). Smartphone based medicine intake scheduler, reminder, and monitor. In *e-Health Networking Applications and Services (Healthcom), 2010 12th IEEE International Conference on.* (pp. 162-168). IEEE.

Chapter 6

# A Blueprint for Designing and Developing M-Health Applications for Diverse Stakeholders Utilizing FHIR

**Mohammed S. Baihan**
*University of Connecticut, USA*

**Christopher Gilman**
*University of Connecticut, USA*

**Yaira K. Rivera Sánchez**
*University of Connecticut, USA*

**Steven A. Demurjian**
*University of Connecticut, USA*

**Xian Shao**
*University of Connecticut, USA*

**Thomas P. Agresta**
*University of Connecticut Health Center, USA*

## ABSTRACT

*FHIR standard is designed to enable interoperability and integration with the newest and adopted technologies by the industry. This chapter presents a number of blueprints for the design and development of FHIR servers that enable the integration between HIT systems with m-health applications via FHIR. Each blueprint is based on the location that FHIR servers can be placed with respect to the components of the m-health application (UI, API, server) or a HIT system in order to define and design the necessary infrastructure to facilitate the exchange of information via FHIR. To demonstrate the feasibility of the work, this chapter utilizes the Connecticut concussion tracker (CT2) m-health application as a proof-of-concept prototype that fully illustrates the blueprints of the design and development steps that are involved. The blueprints can be applied to any m-health application and are informative and instructional for medical stakeholders, researchers, and developers.*

DOI: 10.4018/978-1-5225-5036-5.ch006

## INTRODUCTION

The need to develop mobile applications and services has dramatically increased in the marketplace, with the Gartner group forecasting the business demand for new and diverse mobile applications by the end of 2017 (Moore, 2015) will grow five times larger than the ability of a typical IT organization to deliver. There is an estimate that 2.1 billion mobile phone devices will be sold by 2019, which will increase the demand for new applications with a high performance and usability. According to the PEW Research Center (Smith, 2015), the percentage of American adults Smartphone owners has risen from 35% in 2011 to 64% in 2014 and the percentage is expected to increase in the following years. Moreover, about 62% of Smartphone owners use their phones to keep track of their electronic health records. Since mobile phones are portable and more convenient for typical users, these phones become a dominant way for people to access many services in most governmental and industrial sectors.

In the domain of healthcare, there has been an explosion of mobile health (mHealth) applications for patients (Rickwood, Kleinrock, Núñez-Gaviria, & Sakhrani, 2013) and medical providers (e.g., physicians, nurses, therapists, technicians, specialists, home health aides, etc.) (University of California San Francisco Library, 2016). More and more patients want to utilize a mobile device and mHealth applications to monitor and track his/ her health conditions and fitness. Currently, there are many applications for pharmacies and organizing medications such as myCVS (CVS Pharmacy, 2016), MEDWatcher (MEDWATCHER, 2016), Drugs.com Medication guide and Pill Identifier Applications, (Drugs.com, 2016) etc. For patients, there are also personal health record (PHR) applications such as CAPZULE PHR, (Webahn Incorporation, 2016) MTBC PHR, (MTBC, 2016) suite of WebMD Applications, (WebMD, 2016) etc., and fitness applications such as Apple's HealthKit app (Apple, 2016) and the Google Fit fitness tracker. (Google, 2016) In addition, medical providers seek to access electronic patient data in systems at medical offices, clinics, hospitals, etc., via mHealth applications and also to electronically submit prescriptions.

Collectively, patients and medical providers also desire to utilize the mHealth applications to access different health information technology (HIT) systems that maintain important medical information such as laboratory testing results (Quest Diagnostics, 2016), images and imaging reports (e.g., X-rays, MRIs, Ultrasounds, etc.) (Funt, 2016), etc., to ensure that all of the necessary information is collected for patient care. Examples of HIT systems include: electronic medical records (EMR), personal health records (PHR), pharmacy systems, etc. Enabling mHealth applications to access these HIT systems requires a practical way to send/receive related medical information to/from multiple HIT systems to an mHealth application. However, since each HIT system often requires community developers to access such a system using different formats (i.e., web services, cloud services, Application Programming Interface (API), etc.) and each system identifies medical concepts in different ways, the healthcare data access and health information exchange (HIE) processes become challenging integration problems which may result in increasing healthcare costs (Lamprinakos, Georgios C.; Mousas, Aziz S.; Kapsalis, Andreas P.; Kaklamani, Dimitra I.; Venieris, Iakovos S.; Boufis, Anastasis D.; Karmiris, Panagiotis D.; Mantzouratos, Spyros G., 2014). To solve this problem there is a need for a framework which will reduce such costs (Walker, Pan, Johnston, & Adler-Milstein, 2005), and for the purposes of this chapter, the means for an mHealth application to easily access health/ fitness data from multiple HIT systems.

In support of the interoperability and exchange of health care data, the international Health Level 7 (HL7) (Health Level 7, 2016) organization has taken a leadership role for standards to allow the integration, sharing, and exchange of electronical healthcare data. Specifically, HL7 organization has provided health information exchange standards including: HL7 Version 2, (Health Level 7, HL7 Version 2, 2016) HL7 Version 3 (Health Level 7, HL7 Version 3, 2016), the Clinical Document Architecture (CDA), (Health Level 7, Clinical Document Architecture, 2016) and HL7 Fast Healthcare Interoperability Resources (HL7 FHIR). (Health Level 7, Fast Health Interoperable Resources, 2016) The HL7 V2 standard released in 1989, the most widely adopted interoperability standard in the world, lacked the tools, services, and technologies to satisfy evolving interoperability requirements of state-of-the-art healthcare systems. HL7 V3 was released in 2005, to address V2 deficiencies and introduced concepts that increased the complexity of implementing HL7 V3 and has not been adopted by the industry. The HL7 Fast Healthcare Interoperability Resources (FHIR) was introduced as a first draft in 2011 and is designed to enable interoperability and integration with the newest and adopted technologies by the industry with a particular focus on making healthcare data easily available to mHealth applications via application programming interfaces (API). Specifically, FHIR has adopted the Representational State Transfer (REST) (Fielding, 2000) style to represent all of the entities and procedures in the healthcare setting as FHIR Resources such as Patient, Medication, and Observation (Bender & Sartipi, 2013) that logically partition and abstract the HL7 standard into 90+ resources. To access these Resources, the FHIR API provides a RESTful-based standard that is lightweight and is reasonable to be implemented by mobile devices that provide limited storage and processing capabilities (Mulligan & Gra, 2009).

This chapter presents a number of blueprints for the design and development of FHIR servers that enable the integration between HIT systems and mHealth applications using the FHIR standard. This greatly simplifies the programming complexity and facilitates the ability of mHealth apps to more easily utilize multiple heterogeneous platforms. To demonstrate the feasibility of our work, the chapter utilizes the Connecticut Concussion Tracker (CT²) mHealth application that has been developed as a joint effort between the Departments of Physiology and Neurobiology, and Computer Science & Engineering at the University of Connecticut, in collaboration with faculty in the Schools of Nursing and Medicine. CT² was developed in support of a newly passed law to track concussions for school children (kindergarten through high school) in Connecticut. (Senate and House of Representatives in General, 2014) The CT² mHealth application can be linked via FHIR to a back-end repository that includes both OpenEMR (OEMR, 2016) and OpenMRS (OpenMRS Incorporation, 2016) to represent the clinical repository for students with concussions. However, in this chapter only OpenEMR will be utilized for the purpose of the demonstration of our design and development blueprints.

Our work in this chapter highlights our design and development efforts that serve as blueprints for other stakeholders and that utilize FHIR as a bridge from the CT² mHealth app to OpenEMR with the ability to plug in different EMRs targeting a diverse set of stakeholders: parent/guardians and coaches that do limited reporting via the app at athletic events; athletic trainers that do reporting and basic symptom assessment at athletic events and can monitor the students while at school or at athletic events; nurses that have the most ability to track, modify, and update information on all students in the school; and, administrative staff that have access to summary data (e.g. who has concussions and how many students with concussion). The CT² mHealth app supports role-based access control (RBAC) in a mobile setting (K. Rivera Sánchez, Y.; Demurjian, S.; Conover, J.; Agresta, T.; Shao, X.; Diamond, Michael, 2016) that allows privileges established by the information owner to be defined for users by role, thereby allowing the mobile application to be customized to deliver only authorized information and defined view and/or modify capabilities to the different stakeholders (parents, athletic trainers, coaches, nurses, admins, etc.).

The chapter provides a number of blueprints for the design and development of FHIR servers in which an mHealth application can interact with multiple HIT systems via FHIR through the design, implementation, and usage of FHIR servers. A *FHIR server* is defined to provide a set of RESTful CRUD services to access a particular HIT system and to make calls to the API of the HIT that retrieve data that can then be packaged as FHIR resources. A *FHIR client* is defined for a mobile application that seeks to access Resources from FHIR servers of HIT systems, take the Resources, and convert them into a form that the mobile app can process. The chapter proposes a set of blueprints that differ in the usage and location of FHIR servers with respect to the components of the mHealth application (UI, API, Server) or a HIT system in order to define and design the necessary infrastructure to facilitate the exchange of information via FHIR. One blueprint defines a FHIR server for each HIT which involves identifying the HIT system data items to be sent/ received via the HIT's API and designing an HIT FHIR server to facilitate the exchange that maps the HIT data items to FHIR Resources. A second blueprint defines a FHIR server for the mHealth application, that enables a direct access to its database, which involves identifying the mHealth data items to be sent/received via the mHealth database, and designing an mHealth FHIR server to facilitate the exchange that maps the mHealth data items to FHIR Resources with new FHIR LOAD and STORE RESTful services to support the exchange of the data to/from the mHealth database and the HIT database. A third blueprint defines a FHIR server for the mHealth application, that provides a direct access to its RESTful API, which involves identifying the mHealth data items to be sent/received via the mHealth database and designing an mHealth FHIR server to facilitate the exchange to the FHIR server of one or more HIT systems. A forth blueprint defines a FHIR server for the mHealth application, that uses HIT database as a repository, which involves identifying the mHealth data items to be sent/received via the mHealth app and redesigning the mHealth RESRful API to implement FHIR server to facilitate the exchange to the FHIR server of one or more HIT systems. Note that there are different combinations of these blueprints that can be utilized depending on the configuration of the mobile app with a server and/ or database in a tiered architecture. These blueprints while applied to the $CT^2$ mHealth application are generalizable to any mHealth application and provide a detailed explanation of the processes involved when attempting to integrate an mHealth app with FHIR that can be utilized by other stakeholders.

One main contribution of the chapter are the blueprints of the design and development process that involves the assessment of the mHealth app data and the selection of relevant FHIR resources that are necessary to allow the data entered/managed by mHealth app to be sent/received via FHIR to HIT systems. To demonstrate, we explain the mapping of the concussion data of the $CT^2$ mHealth app to FHIR resources that are then storable in OpenEMR. For example, the FHIR Patient resource can track the concussion incident and associated data for each student. To track concussion data on a student, possible FHIR resources are: the CarePlan resource for basic information, the Condition resource to track the concussion event, the Observation resource to track symptoms, and the Encounter resource to track the different times the nurse makes changes as the concussion is tracked over time. The selection of resources and the mapping of concussion data establish FHIR as middle layer to the $CT^2$ mHealth app which only interacts via FHIR effectively hiding OpenEMR at the backend.

The remainder of this chapter has five sections. The *Background and Motivation* section provides materials on FHIR resources from a development point of view, and related efforts on healthcare systems integration using FHIR. The *Design and Development of FHIR Interoperable Blueprints* section details four blueprints of design and development processes that can link an mHealth application via FHIR to multiple HIT systems via a combination of FHIR servers. The *CT2 mHealth Application and FHIR* section presents a proof-of-concept prototype utilizing the $CT^2$ mHealth concussion app and fully illustrates the blueprints of the design and development steps that are involved. The *Future Trends* section explores the potential future trends that may have an impact on designing healthcare systems with a review of the rapidly growing research and development efforts in FHIR such as Smart on FHIR (Mandel, Kreda, Mandl, Kohane, & Ramoni, 2016), SMART on FHIR Genomics (Alterovitz, Gil; Warner, Jeremy; Zhang, Peijin; Chen, Yishen; Ullman-Cullere, Mollie; Kreda, David; Kohane, Isaac S., 2015), and HEART profile for FHIR (Health Relationship Trust Working Group, 2016). Finally, the *Conclusion* section summarizes the chapter.

## BACKGROUND AND MOTIVATION

This section provides both background and motivation in two different areas. The first area briefly reviews the FHIR framework with a focus on an explanation of FHIR resources from a development point of view to serve as a background for the proposed guideline to design and develop FHIR-based extensions. The second area motivates and presents two related works in the literature that explain alternative ways that FHIR can be implemented to integrate healthcare systems and/or applications in different settings. This area also discusses the deficiencies of the related works and defines the main contributions of this chapter as a further motivation.

The first area reviews the FHIR framework that is primarily structured around the concept of FHIR resources (Health Level 7, Fast Health Interoperable Resources, 2016) which are the data elements and associated application programmer interfaces (API) that can be leveraged for exchanging healthcare information, particularly between mobile applications and HIT systems. FHIR Resources, the main building block in FHIR, can hold any type of information that FHIR deals with to be exchanged from one system to another. FHIR provides different type of such Resources to be utilized by healthcare systems and applications for different purposes. For example, an application may use the Patient resource to store and exchange information about patients back and forth with different HIT systems. All FHIR resources have five main properties in common: a unique URL for identification purposes; common metadata; a human readable section; a number of predefined data elements; and an extension element that enables a system to add new data elements. FHIR provides three formats: UML for a diagrammatic representation of the resource, XML that is the HL7 schema of the resource, and JSON to facilitate a programmatic exchange via a RSETful API. FHIR supports 93 different resource types such as Patient, Medication, and Observation. Figure 1 shows an example of a Patient resource represented in the JSON format. FHIR supports a number of REST API services to enable a system to retrieve and modify data in the Resources. The main five services are: *Create* to add a new instance of a resource; *Read* to retrieve an existing instance of a resource; *Update* to manipulate data in an existing instance of a resource; *Delete* to remove an existing instance of a resource; and, *Search* to retrieve all existing instances of a resource.

The second area reviews two efforts that illustrate FHIR design and implementation: enabling better interoperability for healthcare (Kasthurirathne, Mamlin, Kumara, Grieve, & Biondich, 2015) and applying FHIR in an integrated health monitoring system (Franz, Schuler, & Kraus, 2015). The work in (Kasthurirathne, Mamlin, Kumara, Grieve, & Biondich, 2015) provided a new API module for OpenMRS system that has been built using FHIR. The processes of designing and developing the OpenMRS FHIR API includes: design a framework that assists in adding FHIR-based API for OpenMRS; select a third party FHIR library to implement FHIR resources creation and validation; develop a FHIR-based API for the OpenMRS system;

*Figure 1. An Example of Patient Resource in JSON*

```json
{
  "resourceType": "Patient",
  "id" : "1",
  "meta" : { "versionId" : "1", }
  "text": { "status": "generated", },
  "identifier": [
   {
     "label": "OpenEMR",
     "system": "http://www.healthorg.org/openemr",
     "value": "10"
   }
  ],
  "name": [
  {"family": ["Levin"],
   "given": ["John" ]
   }
  ],
  "gender": {
  "text": "Male" },
  "birthDate": "1985-02-12",
}
```

and, implement the search service of a number of FHIR resources that are capable of retrieve data from the OpenMRS system. The architecture of the proposed FHIR module consists of two layers: the FHIR web layer which mainly retrieves FHIR resources from the FHIR API layer; and, the FHIR API layer that basically models and validates FHIR resources. The initial prototype of the FHIR controller interacted with the Patient and Observation resources with a middle layer that transitions information to/from OpenMRS.

The work of (Franz, Schuler, & Kraus, 2015) presented an extension to a health monitoring system using FHIR to enable interoperability between medical devices and HIT systems. The health monitoring system consists of an *aggregation manager module* which is a mobile device and a *telehealth service center module* which is a server. These two modules were extended by adding components, which are implemented using FHIR, to enable their integration. The aggregation manager module was extended with two services: FHIROBSMessageSender which sends the measured data as Observation FHIR resource to the telehealth service center module; and, FHIRDORMessageSender that sends DeviceObservationReport FHIR resource to the telehealth service center module. The telehealth service center module was extended with two services: OBSController and DORController which receive Observation and DeviceObservationReport FHIR resources respectively from the aggregation manager module. Although these two works successfully applied FHIR to extend different healthcare systems and make such systems more interoperable, the detailed processes of designing and developing FHIR resources are not clearly explained. Moreover, each of these works discussed only one integration option that was specific to the reported effort. In this chapter, we provide a detailed guideline to design and develop FHIR-based extensions for different integration options, so that healthcare organizations and stakeholders may follow the processes of the proposed guideline to design and develop new FHIR-based extensions quickly and easily.

## DESIGN AND DEVELOPMENT OF FHIR INTEROPERABLE BLUEPRINTS

This section of the chapter explores and examines a number of blueprints of design and development processes that can integrate an mHealth application via FHIR to multiple HIT systems. The intent of this section is to present and explain different architecture options that can be utilized in order to allow an mHealth application to interact with multiple HIT systems via FHIR. The remainder of this section is organized into a three-part discussion. In part one, we explore four issues (*overall architecture, involved technologies, source code availability*, and *allowable access to HIT*) that must be understood for an mHealth application to support a discussion of the options and blueprints. In part two, we examine the different architecture options for integrating an mHealth application to multiple HIT systems via FHIR. Lastly, in part three, we provide a blueprint for each provided architecture option that illustrates the way that the options can be realized using FHIR including the various phases and steps that are required.

### Issues That Impact Interoperability

In the first part of this section, we explore the different characteristics and components of a mobile application and its interaction with multiple HIT systems. There are four issues that are discussed: the *overall architecture* of the mHealth application (i.e. one-tier, two-tier, and three-tier architecture); the *involved technologies* (RESTful APIs, programmatic APIs, database API); the *source code availability* of the mobile app, APIs, server code, or database; and the *allowable access* to the HIT sources (RESTful APIs, programmatic APIs). Each are discussed in turn. The first issue that impacts interoperability choices is the *overall architecture* of the mHealth application (one-tier, two-tier, three-tier). That is, in order to integrate an mHealth app with any HIT system one must understand the mHealth app's architecture. In general, there are three different architectures (i.e. one-tier, two-tier, and three-tier). In the one-tier architecture, the mHealth app would contain all of the components of the system including: user interface (the presentation layer); user request processing (the business layer); and the repository (the data layer). In the two-tier architecture, the mHealth app would have the user interface (the presentation layer) while user request processing (the business layer) and the repository (the data layer) are hosted in a separate server. In the three-tier architecture, the mHealth app would only have the user interface (the presentation layer) with the user request processing (the business layer) hosted by a separate server through an API and the repository (the data layer) hosted in another separate (third) server. Note that the repository in all three cases may in turn interact with another layer but from the perspective of the FHIR integration options this will be hidden. Note also that for the two and three tier options, the middle request processing layer might involve access to multiple separate APIs.

The second issue that impacts the choice of an integration option are the *involved technologies* (programmatic API, repository API, RESTful API, cloud services, etc.). These technologies can be utilized by an mHealth app to make external integration possible. Programmatic API of an application is a set of definitions for functions or methods of that application in which an external application may call an API to perform an application's method without the knowledge of the actual code of such a method. Repository API is similar to the programmatic API, however, the functions or methods of such API perform operations over repository items that may be in a database or some other option. A RESTful API is a set of definitions for methods of a web or mobile application. Such an API is designed based on the REST architecture (Fielding, 2000) which utilizes Hypertext Transfer Protocol (HTTP) requests to interact with the data of a resource. Cloud services are the APIs that define the way that cloud consumers can access and utilize cloud computing resources such as software. These cloud services can be designed using web services such as Representational State Transfer (REST), Simple Object Access Protocol (SOAP), etc.

The third issue that impacts the choice of an integration option is the *source code availability* of the mobile app, API, server, or database. Since an mHealth application can be developed based on different architectures (as described in issue 1), it is crucial to consider the availability of source code of components such as the mobile app, APIs, server, or repository. Specifically, the source code of the mobile app is the code that is used to implement: the user interface component; and the methods that interacting with any external servers. The API's source code is the code that is utilized to map the application's methods to an abstract set of calls that an external source can invoke. The server code is the code that is used to implement the business logic of the application. The repository source code is the source file or database schema and any code that is used to access data in such a repository. Some of the FHIR integration options require access to source code in order to make limited programmatic changes to support the integration. The intent is to try to minimize these changes when attempting to integrate a mHealth app with multiple HITs in order to have little or no impact on existing code.

The fourth and final issue that impacts the choice of an integration option is the allowable access to the HIT sources (RESTful API, programmatic API, repository API, cloud services, etc.) to enable external applications to be integrated with such HIT systems. The ability to integrate these various API and services seamlessly with a FHIR server will be critical to support the different integrations options presented in this chapter. In summary, the exact configuration of each of the four aforementioned issues (*overall architecture, involved technologies, source code availability,* and *allowable access to HIT*) has a direct impact on the different available options that can be utilized via FHIR to integrate a particular mHealth application architecture and multiple HIT systems using FHIR servers.

## mHealth Integration Options

In the second part of this section, we enumerate a number of different *mHealth Integration Options* to allow an mHealth application to send/receive data with multiple HIT systems via FHIR via the creation of FHIR servers. To begin, Figure 2 contains anarchitecture of an mHealth app that includes the app, the app's RESTful API, and the app's repository along with three HIT Systems

*Figure 2. mHealth App and HIT Systems*

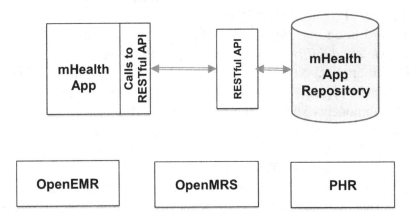

(OpenEMR, OpenMRS, and a PHR such as MTBC (MTBC, 2016)). The different components in Figure 2 will be utilized to define three architectures that illustrate the different ways that the mHealth app can be integrated with the HIT systems based on the four issues previously discussed (*overall architecture, involved technologies, source code availability,* and *allowable access to HIT*). Specifically, we propose: a *Basic Architecture* that includes a FHIR server that works directly with the mHealth App repository and FHIR servers for OpenEMR, OpenMRS, and PHR; an *Alternative Architecture* that includes a FHIR server that works directly with the mHealth App RESTful API and FHIR servers for OpenEMR, OpenMRS, and PHR; and a *Radical Architecture* that removes the repository and has FHIR servers for the mHealth App API, OpenEMR, OpenMRS, and PHR. Note that the HITs that are shown (OpenEMR, OpenMRS, and PHR) are illustrative and in practice a generalized version which have one or more HIT systems.

The *Basic Architecture* option is shown in Figure 3, where the assumption is made that: we have direct access to the mHealth app repository; and, the source codes of mHealth app, mHealth RESTful API, OpenEMR and OpenMRS HIT systems and their APIs are available. In Figure 3, at the bottom, there are FHIR severs (purple ovals) to load/store data from OpenEMR, OpenMRS and PHR (named OpenEMR.FHIR, OpenMRS.FHIR, and PHR.FHIR) using their APIs (a third tier) into selected FHIR Resources; and a mHealth.FHIR server to load/store data from the mHealth repository, at the top of Figure 3. Basically, each HIT systems requires a FHIR server (e.g., OpenEMR.FHIR) to extract data to/from HIT via FHIR resources that in turn interacts with the mHealth.FHIR server of the mHealth App repository. Interactions:

*Figure 3. Basic Architecture with Direct Database Access*

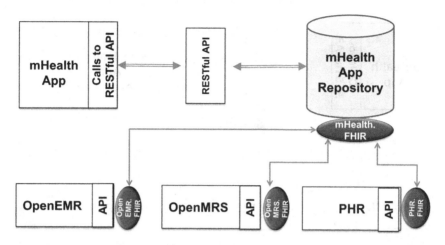

from the mHealth app via its RESTful API are not impacted; and from the mHealth RESTful API to the mHealth repository are not changed as well. However, to enable the mHealth app to take advantage of HIT systems two new FHIR services mHealth.FHIR.LOAD and mHealth.FHIR.STORE are proposed. The mHealth.FHIR.LOAD service will retrieve all of the data from OpenEMR, OpenMRS, or the PHR in the FHIR format. This mHealth.FHIR. LOAD service will take the JSON FHIR from the HIT.FHIR (e.g., OpenEMR. FHIR) server and add them into the mHealth repository via an mHealth FHIR service, which converts the FHIR format into mHealth repository format. This will allow all of the mHealth RESTful API calls to use this temporary data. The mHealth.FHIR.STORE service will grab the data from the mHelath repository, via an mHealth FHIR service, which coverts mHelath repository format into FHIR format and adds them into the OpenEMR, OpenMRS, or the PHR repository. The mHealth.FHIR.LOAD and mHealth.FHIR.STORE services require source code availability of the repository in order to make the needed calls to stage data back and forth from HIT sources. Note that the mHealth.FHIR.LOAD and mHealth.FHIR.STORE services may also be periodically called to ensure that the repositories at both sides are updated. In this way, the mHelath app, API, and repository are not modified.

In the second option, shown in Figure 4, the situation is similar to the basic option in Figure 3, except that there is no direct access to the mHealth app repository. So the mHealth.FHIR server on the mHealth side is moved to directly interact with the mHealth RESTful API. There are still the HIT. FHIR servers for OpenEMR/OpenMRS/PHR as in Figure 3. In this option,

*Figure 4. Alternative Architecture with mHealth RESTful API Access*

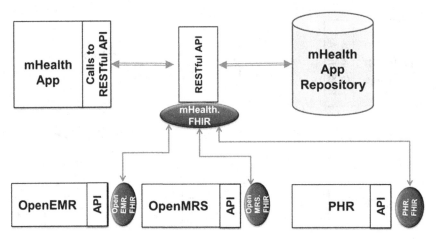

the mHealth App continues to use the mHealth RESTful API without change, however, the mHealth.FHIR.LOAD and mHealth.FHIR.STORE services now become part of the mHealth RESTful API. That is, each mHealth.FHIR. READ service of the mHealth RESTful API first calls the mHealth.FHIR. LOAD service, which takes an id of the queried instance and: retrieves the related data from OpenEMR, OpenMRS, or PHR via their FHIR server; and adds retrieved data into the mHealth repository via another mHealth FHIR API service (i.e. a mHealth.FHIR.CREATE service). This requires slight programmatic changes and source code availability (third issue of prior section). After that, the mHealth.FHIR.READ service of the mHealth RESTful API will retrieve the related data from the mHealth repository (which is updated with the new data from the HIT system). Similarly, each mHealth.FHIR.CREATE service of the mHealth RESTful API first adds the related data into the mHealth repository. After that, the mHealth.FHIR. CREATE service of the mHealth RESTful API calls the STORE service, which takes the newly added data from the mHealth repository via another mHealth.FHIR API service (i.e., a mHealth.FHIR.READ service) and adds them into the OpenEMR, OpenMRS, or the PHR database, via their FHIR service. Note that, in this way, the mHelath app and its calls to the mHealth. FHIR.RESTful API are not modified; however, only a single call to either the mHealth.FHIR.LOAD or mHealth.FHIR.STORE services is added to each RESTful API. This requires source code availability of the RESTful API.

In the *Radical Architecture*, shown in Figure 5, the situation is the same as the alternative option of Figure 4, but radically alters the tiers by removing the repository (database). As a result, this option is a more drastic and involves replacing the mHelath repository and having it rely totally on the HIT systems. This option would move and reconfigure all of the mHealth App data so that it could be stored and managed in the HITs. This will require a totally rewrite of the code for the mHealth RESTful API while still keeping the signatures unchanged so as not to impact the mHealth app. In this case, every rewritten mHealth RESTful API service will implement a mHealth.FHIR service to directly call OpenEMR.FHIR, OpenMRS.FHIR, or PHR.FHIR as required to load/store data as needed. In the Radical Architecture, the services defined are: mHealth.FHIR.CREATE, mHealth.FHIR.READ, mHealth.FHIR.UPDATE, and mHealth.FHIR.DELETE. Source code availability and changing the APIs may be required. This approach is clearly time and effort prohibitive.

## Integration Steps and Processes

The third part of this section involves a discussion of the steps and processes that are necessary to develop the various FHIR servers in Figures 3, 4, and 5 to serve as blueprints for the integration of a mHealth application, via a mHealth.FHIR server that integrates with the mHealth RESTful API, with multiple HIT systems and a HIT.FHIR server that integrates with the APIs of OpenEMR, OpenMRS, and PHR. This essentially functions as guideline

*Figure 5. Radical Architecture without a Database*

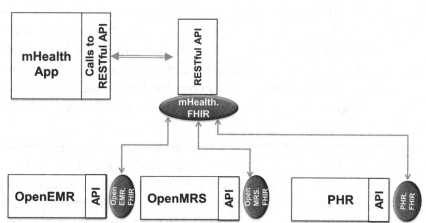

or blueprints for stakeholders of the process to integrate an mHealth app with multiple HIT systems via FHIR using FHIR servers. This section details the blueprints for the Basic (Figure 3), Alternative (Figure 4), and Radical (Figure 5) architectures; all three of these architectures blueprints share the common HIT.FHIR blueprint which involves defining the HIT system data items to be sent/received and designing a HIT.FHIR server to facilitate the exchange. The three architectures have their own specific needs, namely, the mHealth.FHIR server required at the app side Repository in Figure 3, the mHealth.FHIR server in Figure 4, and rewriting the mHealth RESTful API in Figure 5 with a mHealth.FHIR server.

To begin, the common *HIT FHIR Blueprint* involves defining the HIT system data items to be sent/received back and forth via a set of Identified FHIR Resources to another FHIR server or client, and designing a HIT FHIR server (HIT.FHIR) with a RESTful API to facilitate the exchange. The processes of each step are described below:

1. Define the HIT system data items (i.e., for the HIT repositories in Figures 3, 4, and 5) that are needed to be exchanged to/from the mHealth app. This step consists of four sub-steps:
   a. Identify each single candidate data item, e.g., "patient name" table field in the HIT repository that is accessible via an HIT API.
   b. For each candidate data item:
      i. Provide a short and clear item name: by reviewing the FHIR resources, identify a FHIR resource, and map the candidate data item to the most comparable data item of the identified FHIR Resource.
      ii. For the candidate data item, if there is no similar item's name for the identified FHIR resource, identify an item of a FHIR resource that has the same datatype as the candidate data item.
      iii. Provide a brief description that explains the mapping for the case where there is a comparable FHIR data item and more importantly, the case where there is only a comparable FHIR data type.
   c. Group multiple related HIT system data items (e.g., patient name and patient gender) into a separate and distinct data entity (e.g. patient entity). This would make mapping to an Identified FHIR Resource clearer by finding the most similar FHIR resource's name.
   d. End Result: A set of *Identified FHIR Resources* that map to the HIT data entities and items.

2.  Design an HIT.FHIR server in front of the HIT system API in two sub-steps:

    a.  A HIT.FHIR server is designed for all of the Identified FHIR Resources in Step 1d that defines a FHIR API that has CRUD operations for all of the Identified FHIR Resources and interacts with the HIT API.

    b.  Create Classes and CRUD services for all of the Identified FHIR Resources for the HIT.

        i.  Create an HIT.FHIR.Controller class that receives requests from mHealth app (or any other system) and forwards each request to the appropriate Identified FHIR Resource class based on the universally unique identifier (UUID) of an Identified FHIR Resource.

        ii.  Create a class for each Identified FHIR Resource that receives requests from the FHIR controller class and performs the requested CRUD service. This class is defined for each Identified FHIR Resource as HIT.FHIR.IFRCName where IFCRName is the Identified FHIR Resource Class name. This class implements four main CRUD services:

        iii.  A HIT.FHIR.IFRCName.Create service that stores an instance of a FHIR resource from an external call from another FHIR server to create and store new data into the HIT repository. This service takes the data in as a FHIR Resource and then converts the data into a format that can be stored in the HIT repository via a call to one or more HIT API services. This effectively will store FHIR Resource data into the HIT repository. For example, OpenEMR.FHIR.Patient (the Patient FHIR Resource) would call the service of an OpenEMR API that stores the data into the Patient_data table of OpenEMR's MySQL database.

        iv.  A HIT.FHIR.IFRCName.Read service that is a request for an instance of a FHIR resource from an external call from another FHIR server that to read existing data from the HIT repository. This service takes the request for a FHIR Resource that will require a call to one or more HIT API services to retrieve the data from the HIT and create an instance of an Identified FHIR Resource to send back. For example, OpenEMR.FHIR. Patient (the Patient FHIR Resource) would call the service of an OpenEMR API that reads the data from the Patient_data table and perhaps other tables of OpenEMR's MySQL database and creates a FIR HIR ":wHIR Patient instance.

v.    An HIT.FHIR.IFRCName.Update service that receives an instance of a FHIR resource from an external call from another FHIR server to update existing data into the HIT repository. This service takes the data in as a FHIR Resource and then converts the data into a format that can be stored in the HIT repository via a call to one or more HIT API services that update an existing instance.

vi.   A HIT.FHIR.IFRCName.Delete service that receives a request to remove one or more instances (based on the parameters in the request) of a FHIR resource from an external call from another FHIR server to delete existing data from the HIT repository. This service takes the request for a FHIR Resource and interprets the request to call one or more HIT API services to delete instance(s).

Note that in practice, there may be a desire to not implement either HIT. FHIR.IFRCName.Update or HIT.FHIR.IFRCName.Delete services since in electronical medical records, incorrect data is not deleted, but is marked as incorrect. For example, an incorrect laboratory test result assigned to the wrong patient can be marked as not valid.

The *Basic Architecture Blueprint* (Figure 3) allows information from the mHealth repository to be sent/received back and forth via a set of Identified FHIR Resources to another FHIR server or client by designing an mHealth FHIR server (mHealth.FHIR) with a RESTful API to facilitate the exchange. There are three main steps to the blueprint: define the mHealth data items, design the mHealth FHIR server with the LOAD and STORE services, and reuse the HIT FHIR Blueprint.

1.    Define the mHealth data items (i.e., mHealth repository tables' fields in Figure 3) that are needed to be exchanged with an HIT system. This step consists of four sub-steps in which the first three processes are identical to the processes of Step 1 of the HIT FHIR Blueprint with the data items now referring to the mHealth data items as opposed to the HIT data items.

*End Result:* A set of *Identified FHIR Resources* that map to the mHealth data items.

2.  Design the mHealth FHIR server which consists of the mHealth.FHIR. LOAD and mHealth.FHIR.STORE services. This step has two sub-steps.

    a.  A mHealth.FHIR.LOAD service that calls "read" services of an HIT.FHIR to retrieve (in FHIR format) all of the new added data in to HIT repository. Then, the mHealth.FHIR.LOAD service converts the retrieved FHIR resources into a format that can be stored into mHealth repository via mHealth repository API. This read occurs upon startup to initialize the mHealth App repository with information from HITs.

    b.  A mHealth.FHIR.STORE service that calls mHealth repository API to retrieve all of the new added data in mHealth repository, and converts it into FHIR format. Then, the mHealth.FHIR.STORE service simply forwards the converted data to appropriate HIT.FHIR. CREATE services which add the new data into the HIT repository. This store occurs when the mobile app closes to update the HIT repository with information from mHealth repository.

3.  Employ the HIT FHIR Blueprint.

Recall that the Basic architecture has access to the source code of the repository. There may be more than one way to access the repository via Web/cloud services, an API (as with OpenEMR), or by direct programmatic access to the repository (e.g., a MySQL database). As a result, mHealth. FHIR.LOAD and mHealth.FHIR.STORE services would utilize one of these access modes in conjunction with calls to HIT.FHIR CRUD services (e.g., OpenEMR.FHIR.Patient.Read) and take the result of these calls for the identified FHIR resources, and parse and put this information to/from the mHealth repository.

The *Alternative Architecture Blueprint* (Figure 4), also communicates with the common HIT FHIR Blueprint as previously described in the last step of this blueprint. There are four main steps to the Alternative Architecture Blueprint: define the mHealth data items and design the mHealth FHIR server (similar to the one in the Basic Architecture Blueprint), design the LOAD and STORE services, and reuse the HIT FHIR Blueprint. The processes of each step are similar to the ones of the Basic Architecture Blueprint of Figure 3 and are:

1.  Define the mHealth data items (i.e., mHealth repository tables' fields in Figure 4) that are needed to be exchanged with an HIT system. This step consists of four main processes in which the first three processes are identical to the processes of Step 1 of the HIT FHIR Blueprint with

the data items now referring to the mHealth data items as opposed to the HIT data items.

*End Result:* A set of *Identified FHIR Resources* that map to the mHealth data items.

2. Design an mHealth.FHIR server in front of the mHealth RESTful API in two sub-steps:
   a. A mHealth.FHIR server is designed for all of the Identified FHIR Resources in Step 1d that defines a FHIR API that has CRUD operations for all of the Identified FHIR Resources and interacts with the HIT.FHIR server.
   b. Create Classes and CRUD services for all of the Identified FHIR Resources for the mHealth repository.
      i. A mHealth.FHIR.IFRCName. Create service that stores an instance of a FHIR resource from an external call from another FHIR server to create and store new data into the mHealth repository. This takes the data in as a FHIR Resource and then converts the data into a format that can be stored in the mHealth repository via a call to one or more mHealth RESTful API services. This effectively will store FHIR Resource data into the mHealth repository. This would be similar to the OpenEMR example for the HIT.FHIR server.
      ii. A mHealth.FHIR.IFRCName. Read service that is a request for an instance of a FHIR resource from an external call from another FHIR server that to read existing data from the mHealth repository. This takes the request for a FHIR Resource that will require a call to one or more mHealth RESTful API services to retrieve the data from the mHealth repository and create an instance of an Identified FHIR Resource to send back. This would be similar to the OpenEMR example for the HIT.FHIR server.
      iii. An mHealth.FHIR.IFRCName. Update service that receives an instance of a FHIR resource from an external call from another FHIR server to update existing data into the mHealth repository. This takes the data in as a FHIR Resource and then converts the data into a format that can be stored in the mHealth repository via a call to one or more mHealth RESTful API services, updating an existing instance.

iv.   A mHealth.FHIR.IFRCName. Delete service that receives a request to remove one or more instances (based on the parameters in the request) of a FHIR resource from an external call from another FHIR server to delete existing data from the mHealth repository. This takes the request for a FHIR Resource and interprets the request to call one or more mHealth RESTful API services to delete instance(s).

These mHealth.FHIR CRUD services will be called by the mHealth API in order to send information back and forth in a FHIR format that can then be shifted to the HITs via the mHealth.FHIR.LOAD and mHealth.FHIR. STORE operations below.

3.   Design the mHealth.FHIR.LOAD and mHealth.FHIR.STORE services. These two services are located between the mHealth.FHIR server and any HIT system FHIR server and have sub-steps. The HIT.FHIR CRUD services are used to support these functions.

i.   A mHealth.FHIR.LOAD service that calls "read" services of an HIT.FHIR to retrieve (in FHIR format) the new added data into HIT system. Then, the mHealth.FHIR.LOAD service simply forwards the retrieved data to "create" services of mHealth.FHIR which adds the new data into the mHealth repository. This read occurs when the mHealth.FHIR.IFRCName.Read is called to update the mHealth App repository with information from HITs.

ii.   A mHealth.FHIR.STORE service that calls "read" services of the mHealth.FHIR to retrieve (in FHIR format) the new added data in mHealth repository. Then, the mHealth.FHIR.STORE service simply forwards the retrieved data to "create" services of HIT.FHIR which adds the new data into the HIT repository . This store occurs after the mHealth.FHIR.IFRCName.Create is called to update the HIT repository with information from mHealth repository.

4.   Employ the HIT FHIR Blueprint.

Note that in practice, there may be a desire to not implement either mHealth.FHIR.IFRCName.Update or mHealth.FHIR.IFRCName.Delete since in electronical medical records, incorrect data is not deleted, but is marked as incorrect. In this case, we may not want the mHealth app to propagate incorrect data into the HIT systems.

Finally, the *Radical Architecture Blueprint* (Figure 5) has three main steps: define the mHealth data items, redesign the mHealth RESTful API, and communicate the FHIR HIT Blueprint. The processes of these steps are:

1. Define the mHealth data items (see Figure 5) that are needed to be exchanged with an HIT system. This step consists of four main processes in which the first three processes are identical to the processes of Step 1 of the HIT FHIR Blueprint with the data items now referring to the mHealth data items as opposed to the HIT data items.

   *End Result:* A set of *Identified FHIR Resources* that map to the mHealth data items.

2. Redesign the mHealth RESTful API to implement mHealth.FHIR server in two sub-steps:
   a. A mHealth.FHIR server is designed for all of the Identified FHIR Resources in Step 1d that defines a FHIR API that has CRUD operations for all of the Identified FHIR Resources and interacts with the HIT.FHIR.
   b. Create Classes and CRUD services for all of the Identified FHIR Resources for the mHealth app.
      i. A mHealth.FHIR.IFRCName. Create service that receives the new data from the mHealth app, converts it into a format that can be assigned to a FHIR resource, creates an instance of the FHIR resource, and populates the FHIR resource with the converted data. After that, this service calls the HIT. FHIR.IFRCName. Create service with the FHIR resource as a parameter.
      ii. A mHealth.FHIR.IFRCName. Read service that receives the id of a FHIR resource from the mHealth app, invokes the HIT. FHIR.IFRCName. Read service with the id as a parameter. After receiving the result in FHIR format, this service converts the result into a format that can be used by the mHealth app and sends it to the mHealth app.
      iii. An mHealth.FHIR.IFRCName. Update service that is similar to the mHealth.FHIR.IFRCName. Create service, however, this service updates the existing data.

    iv.   A mHealth.FHIR.IFRCName. Delete service that receives the id of a FHIR resource from the mHealth app, calls the HIT. FHIR.IFRCName. Delete service.

3.    Employ the HIT FHIR Blueprint.

Note that in practice, there may be a desire to not invoke either mHealth. FHIR.IFRCName.Update or mHealth.FHIR.IFRCName.Delete services for the same issue discussed above. Also note that there is no need for LOAD and STORE in this Radical option since there is no repository remaining on the mHealth side of Figure 5.

In summary, there are a number of observations to make regarding the FHIR CRUD, LOAD, and STORE services. The CRUD services are defined to manipulate a single FHIR resource that will interact with either the mHealth Repository or the HIT system in order to take information in FHIR format then convert it back and forth into the format of the data items in the Repository/HIT. This will require creating, reading, updating or deleting to/ from the Repository/HIT using the respective API. For the read service on a particular resource, the information is retrieved using services of the API in the native format of the Repository/HIT and converted to either the JSON or XML format of the FHIR resource so that it can be delivered through the FHIR.READ service. For the update service on a particular resource, the resource comes in as either JSON or XML format and the update service would extract out the data items so that they can be assembled to call the appropriate Repository/HIT API services. The create and delete services would work in a similar fashion. The LOAD and STORE services differ in that they will deal with multiple FHIR resources. For STORE, a set of FHIR resources is passed in via a JSON or XML format and these resources are extracted and assembled to allow multiple API services to be called to store the information in the destination format of the Repository or HIT system. For LOAD, multiple API services from the repository/HIT are called to gather information that is then converted and assembled into the appropriate FHIR resources. The resource concept of FHIR facilitates information exchange. However, there is still extraction/conversion required to transition the data from the source to the sharable FHIR format.

## CT² mHealth APPLICATION AND FHIR

This section of this chapter presents a proof-of-concept prototype that demonstrates the ability of a select subset of the Blueprints of the prior section, to enable the integration of an mHealth app with a HIT system using FHIR. In the process, we fully illustrate the application of one of the three architectures blueprints (Basic, Alternative, Radical) and the FHIR HIT blueprint to the Connecticut Concussion Tracker (CT²) mHealth application that has been developed as a joint effort between the Departments of Physiology and Neurobiology, and Computer Science & Engineering at the University of Connecticut, in collaboration with faculty in the Schools of Nursing and Medicine. The CT² app allows the user (e.g., parent/guardian, coach, athletic trainer, school nurse) to report and manage the concussion incidents of students from kindergarten through high school. The CT² mHealth application is linked via FHIR to a back-end repository with OpenEMR (OEMR, 2016) to represent the clinical repository for students with concussions. The remainder of this section is organized into four parts. In part one, we briefly review the CT² mHealth application from a user/functionality perspective. In part two, we detail the off-the-shelf libraries and tools that are employed. In part three, we detail the rational of the chosen architecture option for integrating CT² with OpenEMR using the alternative architecture and defining the two servers: CT².FHIR and OpenEMR.FHIR. Finally, in part four, we apply the guidelines of the previous section to describe the process.

The first part of this section reviews the CT² which is an application for Android and iOS devices that utilizes an API in order to manage its data. The CT² mHealth App contains seven tabs ('Home', 'List', 'Student', 'Cause', 'Symptoms', 'Follow-up', and 'Return') where: the 'Home' tab allows the user to enter a concussion, to retrieve an open case, or to find a student by name; the 'List' tab which contains the list of students the user has permission to view and, for each student gives him/her the option to add a concussion or edit an existing one; the 'Student' tab allows the user to input the student's general information (e.g., name, birthdate, school, and the date of concussion); the 'Cause' tab allows the user to specify how and where the concussion occurred; the 'Symptoms' tab allows users to record the symptoms the student had within 48 hours and other pertinent data; the 'Follow-up' tab allows users to record the status of the student over time; and the 'Return' tab allows users to specify when the student can return to various activities at school. There are four types of users that can interact with the app to report and manage concussion incidents for students. A *School Nurse* user has access to all seven tabs to manage a student's concussion incident from its occurrence to its resolution. An *Athletic Trainer (AT)* user has access to home, list, student, cause, and symptoms tabs to do a limited preliminary assessment if a concussion incident occurs at the event. A *Coach* user has access to home, list, student and cause tabs to report a concussion incident at an athletic event with very limited information on the student. A *Parent/Guardian* user, has access to home, list, student, cause, and symptoms tabs to both report a concussion incident on his/her child while attending the athletic event or to track the current status of his/her children that have ongoing concussions.

The second part of this section discusses off-the-shelf libraries and tools to support the implementation process. Third party FHIR libraries enable a reuse of existing tools that have been developed, tested, and utilized by the healthcare stakeholders and adopting such libraries makes the implementation effort easier. As a result, there is no need to develop FHIR specific modeling and resources; instead, the focus is on implementing the selected integration option. For this demonstration, there are two main third party FHIR libraries that are utilized: the HL7 Application Programming Interface (HAPI) FHIR library that is developed by the HAPI community (HAPI community, 2016), and the FHIR reference implementation (Health Level 7, Health Intersections FHIR Server, 2016) which is built directly from the FHIR specification. The HAPI FHIR library was selected as a FHIR library for the demonstration effort, based on the fact that the HAPI community has a proven track record of long term sustainability and the fact that FHIR standard is already accepted and used by many organizations in the health informatics community.

The third part of this section explains the rationale that dictated the most suitable integration option from the three architectures (Basic, Alternative, Radical) discussed above in this chapter. Among the three architectures (Basic in Figure 3, Alternative in Figure 4, and Radical in Figure 5), the Alternative architecture was chosen, and reconfigured for the $CT^2$ mHealth app as shown in Figure 6. There is a FHIR server for the $CT^2$ RESTful API, $CT^2$.FHIR, and a FHIR server for the OpenEMR API, OpenEMR.FHIR; data is exchanged via FHIR using these two servers. The Alternative Architecture was chosen for a number of reasons. First, we had significant human knowledge of the $CT^2$ mHealth app as two of the co-authors for the chapter are developers of the app and RESTful API and maintain the MySQL database. Second, we had the source code available for the app and RESTful API, and a MySQL database. This meant that we had the ability to do any of the three options,

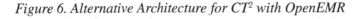

*Figure 6. Alternative Architecture for CT² with OpenEMR*

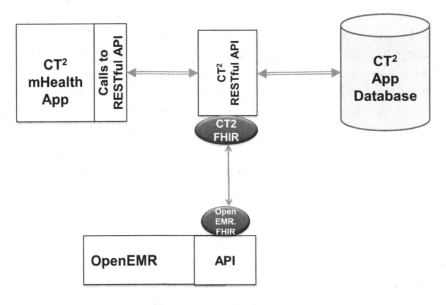

but we chose the Alternative Architecture since it allowed us to maintain the processing and flow of the CT² app through the RESTful API to the database. From the CT² app's perspective, the signatures of the services of the CT² RESTful APIs remained unchanged. From the CT² API's perspective, the interaction with the app and the database remained unchanged. For example, when a user interacts with the CT² app to view and modify a concussion incident for a student, the process transitions from the user request to an API call to a database access to a returned concussion incident. The only change in the process is at the start when a user requests a concussion incident for the student and at the end when a user stores the modified concussion incident for a student; in both cases, the FHIR server of the CT² RESTful API intercepts and retrieves/stores the concussion incident to OpenEMR. When the incident is loaded from OpenEMR via FHIR, a temporary copy is made in the CT² database and all changes that occur via the RESTful API are made to the database on that temporary copy. The final store sends the temporary copy through the CT².FHIR and OpenEMR.FHIR servers to OpenEMR. We decided against the Radical Architecture since we didn't want to make the substantial changes that would be required to migrate all of the information in the CT² database to OpenEMR. This would have included registration information, permissions (who can see/modify which concussion incidents), etc., that would have been difficult to store in OpenEMR.

The fourth part of this section applies the blueprints from the prior section, specifically: the *Alternative Architecture Blueprint* for the mobile app side which utilizes the *HIT FHIR Blueprint* for OpenEMR. For the *Alternative Architecture Blueprint* the four steps can be reformulated as:

1. Define the $CT^2$ mHealth data items from the $CT^2$ that need to be exchanged with OpenEMR via FHIR to yield the Identified FHIR resources for $CT^2$.
2. Design a $CT^2$.FHIR server in front of the $CT^2$ RESTful API.
3. Design $CT^2$.FHIR CRUD services ($CT^2$.FHIR.IFRCName.Create, $CT^2$.FHIR.IFRCName.Read, $CT^2$.FHIR.IFRCName.Update, and $CT^2$.FHIR.IFRCName.Delete) and $CT^2$.FHIR.LOAD and $CT^2$.FHIR.STORE services that extend the $CT^2$ RESTful API so that the exchange via FHIR can occur with OpenEMR.
4. Employ the HIT FHIR Blueprint.

For the *HIT FHIR Blueprint* the two steps can be reformulated as:

1. Define the OpenEMR system data items that are needed to be exchanged to/from the $CT^2$ mHealth app via FHIR to yield the Identified FHIR resources for OpenEMR.
2. Design a OpenEMR.FHIR server in front of the OpenEMR system API.

The main focus for both of these blueprints is in Step 1 of each, to identify the data items that need to be exchanged from each side via FHIR. This will require a designer to understand the correspondence between two sets of information:

- The data items of the $CT^2$ concussion MySQL database and the relevant FHIR resources that can be chosen to store them.
- The data items of the OpenEMR MySQL database and the relevant FHIR resources that can be chosen to store them.

The challenge is to consider these correspondences simultaneously to understand the way that the data items of the concussion app can be mapped via FHIR resources to the data items of OpenEMR. The end result will be a set of Identified FHIR resources that will serve as the common layer to facilitate the exchange of data between $CT^2$ and OpenEMR via FHIR services.

To begin this analysis process, in Step 1 of the *Alternative Architecture Blueprint,* we start by identifying the six key data items of $CT^2$ mHealth that are in six tables of the MySQL Concussion database, namely: the Students table that tracks basic information on students (e.g., demographics, school, etc.); the Incidents table that tracks information on the concussion incident (e.g., when concussion happened, initial symptoms, etc.); the Incident_Locations table that tracks where the concussion occurred (e.g., at school, at sports field, at home, etc.); the Incident_Lingering_Symptoms table that tracks concussion symptoms (e.g., dizzy, nauseous, etc.); the Incident_Updates table that keeps track of all of the major events after the concussion incident (e.g., follow up with physician, return to school, etc.); and, the Incident_Records_Status which records major events and their dependencies. These six tables are shown in Figure 7.

Given the understanding of this information, we can continue the analysis process with Step 2 of the *Alternative Architecture Blueprint* to determine the Identified FHIR Resources that can be utilized to capture the information from Figure 7. To track concussion data on a student we can use the FHIR resources (Health Level 7, Fast Health Interoperable Resources, 2016) as shown in Figure 8. The Identified FHIR Resources are: Patient, Condition, Encounter, EpisodeOfCare, Observation, and Care Plan. Specifically: Patient to track demographic and other basic information on patients (students that

*Figure 7. CT² Data Items of Interest*

| Students |
|---|
| student_id |
| first_name |
| middle_name |
| last_name |
| suffix |
| Email |
| student_number |
| school_id |

| incidents |
|---|
| incident_id |
| incident_reference_id |
| student_id |
| incident_location_id |
| incident_location_details |
| sport_id |
| contact_mechanism_id |
| impact_location_id |
| Removed |
| removed_by_user_id |
| tool_id |
| symptom_comments |
| Date |
| school_id |
| reporting_user_id |
| head_gear_usage |
| parents_notified |
| loss_conciousness |

| incident_updates |
|---|
| follow_up_id |
| incident_id |
| reporting_user_id |
| lingering_symptoms_record _id |
| lingering_description |
| time_resolved |
| diagnosed_by |
| pcs_diagnosis |
| Imaging |
| follow_up_comments |
| days_absent |
| scheduled_modified |
| plan_504 |
| rtl_date |
| rtp_date |
| Date |

| incident_records_status |
|---|
| record_id |
| incident_id |
| follow_up_id |
| user_id |
| date |
| operation_type_id |
| closed |
| updated |

| incident_lingering_symptoms |
|---|
| record_id |
| symptom_id |

| incident_locations |
|---|
| location_id |
| title |
| description |

*Figure 8. FHIR Resources of Interest*

| Patient |
| --- |
| Id |
| name.given |
| name.given |
| name.family |
| name.suffix |
| Telecom |
| Identifier |
| managingOrganization |

| Condition |
| --- |
| id |
| Code |
| Patient.reference |
| Encounter.id |
| Notes |
| category |
| Evidence.id |
| bodySite |
| clinicalStatus |
| Asserter |
| Abatement |
| evidence.detail |
| dateRecorded |
| identifier |
| Encounter.reference |
| Evidence.detail |
| Evidence.FormatComment |
| Evidence.hashCode |

| CarePlan |
| --- |
| Id |
| Subject.id |
| Author |
| Activity.detail.reasonReference |
| Description |
| Quantity |
| Participant.member |
| Activity.detail.category |
| Activity.detail.code |
| Activity.detail.description |
| activity.detail.dailyAmount |
| Activity.detail.scheduled.scheduledString |
| Status |
| activity.detail.scheduled.scheduledTiming |
| Period |
| Modified |

| EpisodeOfCare |
| --- |
| Id |
| condition.id |
| text |
| patient.id |
| period.start |
| type |
| status |
| meta |

| Observation |
| --- |
| id |
| Encounter.id |
| Subject.id |
| Performer.id |
| issued |
| related.type |
| status |
| value |

| Encounter |
| --- |
| Id |
| location |
| reason |

suffer concussions); Condition to track a medical condition, in our case a concussion; Encounter to track the different times that changes are made, in our case, as the concussion incident is tracked over time; EpisodeofCare to keep track of different events for (students); Observation to track symptoms of patients (students); and CarePlan to track the planned treatment for a condition (concussion). Examining the MySQL tables of the $CT^2$ database in comparison to the aforementioned FHIR resources, we can establish a correspondence or mapping between them as shown in Figure 9. In the mapping: students ⇔ Patient; incidents ⇔ Condition; incident_updates ⇔ CarePlan; incident_records_status ⇔ EpisodeOfCare; incident_lingering_symptoms ⇔ Observations; and incident_locations⇔ Encounter.

Now, let's turn the discussion to Steps 1 and 2 of the *HIT FHIR Blueprint* that involves an analogous process to Figures 7, 8, and 9, with the data items of OpenEMR. Since we have already arrived at the FHIR resources needed for mapping (Figure 8), we can reuse the aforementioned Identified FHIR Resources to assist in the identification of the appropriate six data items in OpenEMR in Figure 10, namely: the Patient_Data table that tracks patient

*Figure 9. Mapping from CT² to/from FHIR*

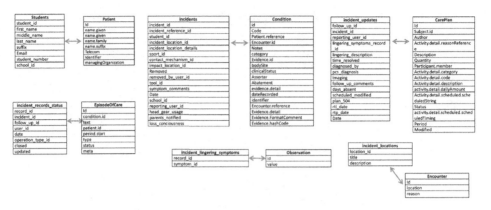

*Figure 10. The OpenEMR Data Items of Interest*

| Patient_data |
|---|
| Pid |
| Fname |
| Mname |
| Lname |
| Title |
| Email |
| Pubpid |
| referrerID |

| Lists |
|---|
| Id |
| Title |
| Pid |
| injury_type |
| Extrainfo |
| Activity |
| injury_grade |
| injury_part |
| Occurance |
| User |
| reinjury_id |
| Comments |
| Begdate |
| Destination |
| Referredby |
| Type |
| Classification |
| Diagnosis |

| transactions |
|---|
| Id |
| title |
| User |
| refer_related_code |
| refer_diag |
| refer_risk_level |
| refer_external |
| reply_services |
| reply_from |
| reply_recommend |
| refer_from |
| reply_findings |
| reply_init_diag |
| refer_reply_date |
| reply_date |
| Date |

| procedure_report |
|---|
| procedure_report_id |
| procedure_order_id |
| procedure_order_seq |
| specimen_num |
| date_report |
| report_notes |
| report_status |
| review_status |

| procedure_order_code |
|---|
| procedure_order_id |
| procedure_order_seq |

| form_encounter |
|---|
| id |
| facility |
| reason |

(student) demographic data; the Lists table that tracks issues related to medical problems, etc. (concussion medical problem); the Form_Encounter table that tracks the event involved with the patient visiting (student seeing nurse); the Procedure_Report that tracks various procedures on patients (actions on students); the Procedure_Order_Code table that tracks different codes associated with procedures; and, the Transactions table that tracks historical events (incident updates on students). These six items correspond to the FHIR Resources as shown in Figure 11. In the mapping: Patient_data ⟺ Patient; Lists

*Figure 11. Mapping from OpenEMR to/from FHIR*

| Patient_data |
| --- |
| Pid |
| Fname |
| Mname |
| Lname |
| Title |
| Email |
| Pubpid |
| referrerID |

| Patient |
| --- |
| Id |
| name.given |
| name.given |
| name.family |
| name.suffix |
| Telecom |
| Identifier |
| managingOrganization |

| Lists |
| --- |
| Id |
| Title |
| Pid |
| injury_type |
| Extrainfo |
| Activity |
| injury_grade |
| injury_part |
| Occurance |
| User |
| reinjury_id |
| Comments |
| Begdate |
| Destination |
| Referredby |
| Type |
| Classification |
| Diagnosis |

| Condition |
| --- |
| id |
| Code |
| Patient.reference |
| Encounter.id |
| Notes |
| category |
| Evidence.id |
| bodySite |
| clinicalStatus |
| Asserter |
| Abatement |
| evidence.detail |
| dateRecorded |
| identifier |
| Encounter.reference |
| Evidence.detail |
| Evidence.FormatComment |
| Evidence.hashCode |

| transactions |
| --- |
| Id |
| User |
| refer_related_co |
| de |
| refer_diag |
| refer_risk_level |
| refer_external |
| reply_services |
| reply_from |
| reply_recommen |
| d |
| refer_from |
| reply_findings |
| reply_init_diag |
| refer_reply_date |
| reply_date |
| Date |

| CarePlan |
| --- |
| Id |
| Subject id |
| Author |
| Activity.detail.reasonReferenc e |
| Description |
| Quantity |
| Participant.member |
| Activity.detail.category |
| Activity.detail.code |
| Activity.detail.description |
| activity.detail.dailyAmount |
| Activity.detail.scheduled.sche duledString |
| Status |
| activity.detail.scheduled.sched uledTiming |
| Period |
| Modified |

| procedure_report |
| --- |
| procedure_report_id |
| procedure_order_id |
| procedure_order_seq |
| specimen_num |
| date_report |
| report_notes |
| report_status |
| review_status |

| EpisodeOfCare |
| --- |
| Id |
| condition.id |
| text |
| patient.id |
| period.start |
| type |
| status |
| meta |

| procedure_order_code |
| --- |
| procedure_order_id |
| procedure_order_seq |

| Observation |
| --- |
| Id |
| value |

| form_encounter |
| --- |
| id |
| facility |
| reason |

| Encounter |
| --- |
| Id |
| location |
| reason |

⇔ Condition; transactions ⇔ CarePlan; procedure_report ⇔ EpisodeOfCare; procedure_order_code ⇔ Observations; and form_encounter ⇔ Encounter.

The last step of the *HIT FHIR Blueprint* is the creation of the OpenEMR. FHIR server. As described in the *HIT FHIR Blueprint* and based on the selected FHIR resources in the provisos steps, we created a FHIR controller class which receives requests from the CT² mHealth app and sends the request to the appropriate OpenEMR FHIR resource class along with any parameters; and six OpenEMR Identified FHIR Resources (i.e., Patient, Condition, CarePlan, EpisodeOfCare, Observation, and Encounter) as shown in the bottom of Figure 12. For each of these OpenEMR FHIR resources classes, we defined: OpenEMR.FHIR.IFRCName.Create and OpenEMR. FHIR.IFRCName.Read). The OpenEMR.FHIR.IFRCName.Create service receives from the CT2 mHealth app an instance of a FHIR resource that involves new data, of a specific class, converts the data into a format that can be stored in OpenEMR system, and sends the converted data to a create service of OpenEMR system API that will store the data into the OpenEMR system database. The OpenEMR.FHIR.IFRCName.Read service retrieves data from the OpenEMR system database via a read service of OpenEMR system API, creates a new instance of the specific FHIR resource class, and converts the retrieved data into a format that can be assigned to the identified OpenEMR FHIR resource instance. Following that, this service populates the corresponding OpenEMR FHIR resource instance with the converted data, and sends this FHIR resource instance to the CT² mHealth app. This service is also designed to retrieve all of the related data on the specific data item if there are no passed parameters.

*Figure 12. Combined Result of Two Blueprints*

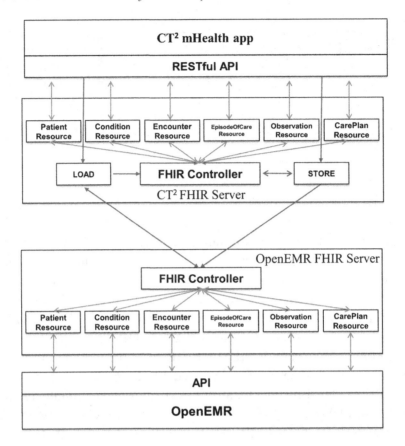

Finally, the remaining step of the *Alternative Architecture Blueprint* is to implement the $CT^2$.FHIR server. As described in the *Alternative Architecture Blueprint* and based on the selected FHIR resources, we created a FHIR controller class which receives requests from the $CT^2$.FHIR.LOAD and $CT^2$.FHIR.STORE services; and sends the request to the appropriate $CT^2$ FHIR resource class along with any parameters; and six $CT^2$ Identified FHIR resources classes (i.e., Patient, Condition, CarePlan, EpisodeOfCare, Observation, and Encounter) as the top of Figure 12 shows. For each of these $CT^2$ FHIR resources classes we created two main CRUD services (i.e. $CT^2$.FHIR.IFRCName.Create and $CT^2$.FHIR.IFRCName.Read); and created $CT^2$.FHIR.LOAD and $CT^2$.FHIR.STORE services. The $CT^2$.FHIR.IFRCName.Create service receives an instance of a FHIR resource with new data, converts the data into a format that can be stored in the $CT^2$ database, and sends the converted data to the $CT^2$ RESTful API (a create service) which stores the data into the $CT^2$ database. The $CT^2$.FHIR.IFRCName.Read service retrieves data from the $CT^2$ database via a $CT^2$ RESTful API (a read service), creates a new instance of related $CT^2$ FHIR resource class, and converts the retrieved data into a format that can be assigned to the $CT^2$ FHIR resource instance. After that, this service populates the $CT^2$ FHIR resource instance with the converted data, and finally sends this FHIR resource instance to the request source. This service also retrieves all of the related data about specific data item if there are no passed parameters. The $CT^2$.FHIR.LOAD service takes an id of the queried $CT^2$.FHIR resource instance, retrieves the related data from the OpenEMR system via OpenEMR.FHIR server, and adds retrieved data into the $CT^2$ database via another $CT^2$ FHIR service (i.e. the $CT^2$.FHIR. IFRCName.Create service). Finally, the $CT^2$.FHIR.STORE service calls $CT^2$. FHIR.IFRCName.Read service to retrieve (in FHIR format) all of the new added data in $CT^2$ database. Then, the $CT^2$.FHIR.STORE service simply sends the retrieved data to "create" services of OpenEMR.FHIR which adds the new data into the OpenEMR system.

## FUTURE TRENDS

This section explores the potential future trends that may support the ability of mobile health (mHealth) applications to interact with multiple HIT systems and trends that can support healthcare IT in general. The discussion is focused on the emerging efforts in leveraging and extending FHIR to support healthcare systems with a review of the rapidly growing research and development efforts in FHIR that include: SMART on FHIR, SMART on FHIR Genomics, and HEART profile for FHIR. The first effort, the Substitutable Medical Apps and Reusable Technology (SMART) project, was initiated by Harvard Medical School and Boston Children's Hospital with an aim to enable interoperability between medical applications by providing a specification to enable developers in the health informatics community to create medical applications once and deploy them across different HIT systems without rewriting the application code for each HIT systems (Mandl, et al., 2012). SMART on FHIR (Mandel, Kreda, Mandl, Kohane, & Ramoni, 2016), is a recently released version of SMART that adopts numerous FHIR main features. This includes: FHIR data models, data formats, and API; authorization using OAuth2 (OAuth, 2016); authentication utilizing OpenID connect (OpenID, 2016); SMART profiles that integrate with FHIR profiles; and EHR user interface integration. Specifically, the SMART on FHIR reference platform has been implemented with three main servers: an API server that provides create, read, update, and delete services for all FHIR resources with an implementation of the FHIR search service; an authorization server which is a modified implementation of an open source OAuth2 and OpenID servers; and, an applications server that uses an EHR-like framework for developers to retrieve a list of patient data. By providing this reference platform, SMART on FHIR enables flexibility and innovations and enables systems to grow quickly as user needs change.

SMART on FHIR Genomics (Alterovitz, Gil; Warner, Jeremy; Zhang, Peijin; Chen, Yishen; Ullman-Cullere, Mollie; Kreda, David; Kohane, Isaac S., 2015) is a specification that adds genomic capabilities to FHIR with the intent to integrate genomic and clinical data. The work proposes three new FHIR resource and extension definitions: a Sequence resource for capturing a patient's genetic data; a SequencingLab extension to capture the specific sequencing technique which is utilized to generate sequences; and a GeneticObservation extension to associate a phenotype to variant data. SMART on FHIR Genomics extends the SMART on FHIR platform by adding features that enable developers to bridge between the genomics and clinical communities via one integrated platform, thereby supporting the combination of different sources of genomic and electronic medical record (EMR) clinical data. The end result of such a combination is the ability to develop new types of medical and healthcare applications that can be utilized for precision and personalized medicine.

The HEART Working Group (Health Relationship Trust Working Group, 2016) was formed to develop a unified set of privacy and security specifications that would be able to control authorization to RESTful APIs. As part of this effort, a HEART profile is being proposed that is capable of interacting with various authentication protocols and tools: OAuth 2.0, OpenID Connect, FHIR OAuth 2.0 Scopes, and User-Managed Access. The addition of the OAuth 2.0 protocol to the FHIR standard to prevent privacy and security issues that a FHIR implementation may face would be an important extension to FHIR that further enhances the interoperability of FHIR. The intent is to allow customized access to a set of RESTful health-related data sharing Application Program Interfaces (APIs) that would be capable of controlling access to different portions of the API on a user/role and/or application basis. This extends OAuth 2.0 that had typically focused on the access of a client to a system to a more fine grained security access to control who can utilize which services of an API. To achieve this, the HEART profile for FHIR introduces the concept of scopes to restrict access to different parts of an API. For example, scopes can be utilized to restrict: the type of resource (e.g., Patient, Observation, etc.) to be protected; the type of access to a requested resource (e.g. read, create, and delete) which is essentially the CRUD services that can be invoked; and, the exact part of a resource to be accessed (e.g., user ID and resource ID). A scope value is a composite text that contains: the type of permission, the type of resource, and the type of access to that resource being requested.

## CONCLUSION

In this chapter, a number of blueprints for the design and development of an mHealth application that interacts with multiple HIT systems via FHIR have been presented. The work presented in this chapter demonstrated architecture options to integrate an mHealth application that hides many technical details of different systems and provided the stakeholders of healthcare systems and mHealth applications with different ways to take advantage of all the participating systems. The result are blueprints for the design and development of an mHealth application for diverse stakeholders that leverages the FHIR framework to facilitate interactions with multiple health information technology (HIT) systems. The *Design and Development of FHIR Interoperable Blueprint* section supported this process and discussed four critical issues (overall architecture, involved technologies, source code availability, and allowable access to HIT), introduced three architectures for interoperation (Basic, Alternative, Radical), and presented four blueprints (*Basic Architecture Blueprint, Alternative Architecture Blueprint, Radical Architecture Blueprint* and *HIT FHIR Blueprint*). The blueprints that were then demonstrated for the CT$^2$ mHealth app linked via FHIR to OpenEMR that can be generalized to be applied to any mHealth application, resulting in a discussion that is both informative and instructional for medical stakeholders, researches, and developers. By adopting a lightweight RESTful-based API of the HL7 FHIR standard, the mHealth applications can interact with multiple HIT systems via that common standard. This is expected to enable developers to easily create mHealth applications with many features that are compatible with multiple HIT systems via a common framework (FHIR). To place the work into context, the *Future Trends* section explored research and development efforts in FHIR such as Smart on FHIR, (Mandel, Kreda, Mandl, Kohane, & Ramoni, 2016) SMART on FHIR Genomics, (Alterovitz, Gil; Warner, Jeremy; Zhang, Peijin; Chen, Yishen; Ullman-Cullere, Mollie; Kreda, David; Kohane, Isaac S., 2015) and HEART profile for FHIR (Health Relationship Trust Working Group, 2016).

## REFERENCES

Aitken, M., & Gauntlett, C. (2013). *Patient apps for improved healthcare: from novelty to mainstream*. Parsippany, NJ: IMS Institute for Healthcare Informatics.

Alterovitz, G., Warner, J., Zhang, P., Chen, Y., Ullman-Cullere, M., Kreda, D., & Kohane, I. S. (2015). SMART on FHIR Genomics: Facilitating standardized clinico-genomic apps. *Journal of the American Medical Informatics Association*, 1–6. PMID:26198304

Apple. (2016). *iOS 8 Health*. Retrieved March 17, 2016, from https://www.apple.com/ios/ios8/health/

Bender, D., & Sartipi, K. (2013). HL7 FHIR: An Agile and RESTful approach to healthcare information exchange. In *The 26th IEEE International Symposium on Computer-Based Medical Systems* (pp. 326-331). IEEE.

CVS Pharmacy. (2016). *CVS mHealth*. Retrieved February 13, 2016, from http://www.cvs.com/mobile-cvs

Drugs.com. (2016). *Drugs.com mHealth*. Retrieved March 19, 2016, from http://www.drugs.com/apps/

Fielding, R. T. (2000). *Architectural styles and the design of network-based software architectures* (Doctoral dissertation). Irvine, CA: University of California.

Franz, B., Schuler, A., & Kraus, O. (2015). *Applying FHIR in an Integrated Health Monitoring System*. EJBI.

Funt, S. (2016). *My Imaging Records App*. Retrieved March 22, 2016, from http://myimagingrecords.com/index.html

Google. (2016). *Fitness Tracker App*. Retrieved March 15, 2016, from https://play.google.com/store/apps/details?id=com.realitinc.fitnesstracker

HAPI Community. (2016). *About HAPI*. Retrieved March 23, 2016, from http://hl7api.sourceforge.net/

Health Level 7. (2016a). *About HL7*. Retrieved March 14, 2016, from http://www.hl7.org/

Health Level 7. (2016b). *Clinical Document Architecture*. Retrieved March 15, 2016, from http://www.hl7.org/implement/standards/product_brief.cfm?product_id=7

Health Level 7. (2016c). *Fast Health Interoperable Resources*. Retrieved March 16, 2016, from http://www.hl7.org/implement/standards/fhir/

Health Level 7. (2016d). *Health Intersections FHIR Server*. Retrieved March 08, 2016, from http://fhir2.healthintersections.com.au/open

Health Level 7. (2016e). *HL7 Version 2*. Retrieved March 14, 2016, from http://www.hl7.org/implement/standards/product_brief.cfm?product_id=185

Health Level 7. (2016f). *HL7 Version 3*. Retrieved March 14, 2016, from https://www.hl7.org/implement/standards/product_brief.cfm?product_id=186

Health Relationship Trust Working Group. (2016). *HEART profile for FHIR*. Retrieved March 22, 2016, from http://openid.net/wg/heart/

Kasthurirathne, S. N., Mamlin, B., Kumara, H., Grieve, G., & Biondich, P. (2015). Enabling Better Interoperability for HealthCare: Lessons in Developing a Standards Based Application Programing Interface for Electronic Medical Record Systems. *Journal of Medical Systems*, 1–8. PMID:26446013

Lamprinakos, G. C., Mousas, A. S., Kapsalis, A. P., Kaklamani, D. I., Venieris, I. S., Boufis, A. D., & Mantzouratos, S. G. (2014). *Using FHIR to develop a healthcare mobile application. In Wireless Mobile Communication and Healthcare (Mobihealth)* (pp. 132–135). IEEE.

Mandel, J. C., Kreda, D. A., Mandl, K. D., Kohane, I. S., & Ramoni, R. B. (2016). SMART on FHIR: a standards-based, interoperable apps platform for electronic health records. *Journal of the American Medical Informatics Association*. Retrieved March 25, 2016, from http://docs.smarthealthit.org/

MEDWATCHER. (2016). *MEDWATCHER mHealth*. Retrieved March 18, 2016, from https://medwatcher.org/

Moore, S. (2015). *Gartner Says Demand for Enterprise Mobile Apps Will Outstrip Available Development Capacity Five to One*. Retrieved March 13, 2016, from http://www.gartner.com/newsroom/id/3076817

MTBC. (2016). *MTBC PHR*. Retrieved March 18, 2016, from https://phr.mtbc.com/

Mulligan, G., & Gra, D. (2009). *A comparison of SOAP and REST implementations of a service based interaction independence middleware framework. In The 2009 Winter Simulation Conference (WSC)* (pp. 1423–1432). IEEE.

OAuth. (2016). *About OAuth 2.0*. Retrieved March 06, 2016, from https://oauth.net/2/

OEMR. (2016). *About OpenEMR*. Retrieved March 11, 2016, from http://www.open-emr.org/

Open, I. D. (2016). *About OpenID Connect*. Retrieved March 24, 2016, from http://openid.net/connect/

OpenMRS Incorporation. (2016). *About OpenMRS*. Retrieved March 10, 2016, from http://openmrs.org/

Quest Diagnostics. (2016). *MyQuest Apps*. Retrieved March 20, 2016, from https://myquest.questdiagnostics.com/web/home

Rickwood, S., Kleinrock, M., Núñez-Gaviria, M., & Sakhrani, S. (2013). *The Global Use of Medicines: Outlook through 2017*. Parsippany, NJ: IMS Institute for Healthcare Informatics.

Rivera Sánchez, K. Y., Demurjian, S., Conover, J., Agresta, T., Shao, X., & Diamond, M. (2016). An Approach for Role-Based Access Control in Mobile Applications. In S. Mukherja (Ed.), Mobile Application Development, Usability, and Security. IGI Global.

Senate and House of Representatives in General. (2014). *An act concerning youth athletics and concussions*. Hartford, CT: Author.

Smith, A. (2015). *U.S. Smartphone Use in 2015*. Retrieved January 08, 2016, from http://www.pewinternet.org/2015/04/01/us-smartphone-use-in-2015/

University of California San Francisco Library. (2016). *Mobile Apps for Healthcare Professionals*. Retrieved January 19, 2016, from http://guides. ucsf.edu/c.php?g=100993&p=654826

Walker, J., Pan, E., Johnston, D., & Adler-Milstein, J. (2005). The value of health care information exchange and interoperability. *Health Affairs*, 24. PMID:15659453

Web, M. D. (2016). *WebMD Apps*. Retrieved March 12, 2016, from http:// www.webmd.com/mobile

Webahn Incorporation. (2016). *Single App to Track Health and Wellness of Your Family*. Retrieved March 19, 2016, from https://www.capzule.com/

## KEY TERMS AND DEFINITIONS

**Application Programming Interface (API):** Is a collection of functions, protocols, and tools that enable third party developers to use and extend the functionalities of existing applications.

**Electronic Medical Record (EMR):** Is a digital form that is equivalent to paper-based patient medical data.

**Fast Healthcare Interoperability Resources (FHIR):** Is a specification provided by HL7 that adopts the representational state transfer (REST) style to represent all entities and procedures in the healthcare setting as resources.

**FHIR Resource:** Is the main building block in FHIR that can hold any type of information that FHIR deals with to exchange from one system to another. FHIR resource examples include patient, medication, and observation.

**Health Information Exchange (HIE):** Is the portability of healthcare information electronically across organizations within a region, community, or hospital HIT systems.

**Health Information Technology (HIT) Systems:** Special type of information technology systems that help users in the healthcare domain to provide acceptable level of health services and care.

**Health Level Seven International (HL7):** An organization that develops standards that help health information technology systems developers and designers to manage electronic health data.

**Interoperability:** Is a software feature that enables a variety of HIT systems and applications to communicate, exchange data, and use the information that has been exchanged.

**M-Health Application:** Is a mobile application that is developed to be used by healthcare stakeholders such as patients and medical providers.

**Personal Health Record (PHR):** Is an application utilized by patients to maintain and manage their health information in a private, secure, and confidential environment.

# Chapter 7
# Geo–Location–Based File Security System for Healthcare Data

**Govinda K.**
*VIT University, India*

## ABSTRACT

*Nowadays, a person's medical information is just as important as their financial records as they may include not only names and addresses but also various sensitive data such as their employee details, bank account/credit card information, insurance details, etc. However, this fact is often overlooked when designing a file storage system for storing healthcare data. Storage systems are increasingly subject to attacks, so the security system is quickly becoming a mandatory feature of the data storage systems. For the purpose of security, we are dependent on various methods such as cryptographic techniques, two-step verification, and even biometric scanners. This chapter provides a mechanism to create a secure file storage system that provides two-layer security. The first layer is in the form of a password, through which the file is encrypted at the time of storage, and second is the locations at which the user wants the files to be accessed. Thus, this system would allow a user to access a file only at the locations specified by him/her. Therefore, the objective is to create a system that provides secure file storage based on geo-location information.*

DOI: 10.4018/978-1-5225-5036-5.ch007

# INTRODUCTION

The ways of the healthcare industry have changed significantly over the previous decade, as those who give health related administrations have started moving from paper-based procedures to electronic strategies. Today, it is not unusual to have a specialist enter an exam room with a portable workstation close by rather than use paper based charts. The medicinal services business produces enormous amount of information and those in the field perceive the advantages of consolidating more computerized procedures into their day to day operations such as cost investment funds, expanded effectiveness, and enhanced interchanges, to name a few.

The class of people who work towards obtaining people's sensitive information and misuse it have now become more interested in their healthcare records as it provides them not only with their personal details such as name, address etc., but also other valuable information such as employer details, bank accounts/credit card information. By taking a patient's personal information and medical data, they can illicitly get medical goods and services. The victims are then left to manage the specialists, hospitals, insurance agencies etc. to determine the resulting monetary aftermath. Now and again, the victim can even lose their insurance, bringing about unreasonable out-of-pocket instalments to have their insurance re-established. There is additionally the threat of the true patient's medical records being changed or inaccurate data being inserted as a consequence of abuse or carelessness, which may keep them from getting legitimate treatment.

However, this sensitive nature of healthcare information is often overlooked when designing a file storage system for storing healthcare data. Therefore there is a need to implement secure file storage systems for healthcare data. This security can be authorized by utilizing various cryptographic procedures. Along with the assistance of these procedures the imperative documents can be encrypted and the clients can be given their suitable cryptographic keys.

Two-factor authentication systems have usually joined something you know, for example, a secret key or passphrase, with a second component to expand verification quality: either something you have, (for example, an entrance card or token), or something you are, (for example, biometrics). A supplementary component has recently been added to this to improve validation abilities: "somewhere you are", also called geolocation. Using this feature in a multi-element verification system, we can limit remote access of documents to specific trusted areas.

Geolocation is a term used in information systems security circles to extrapolate the geographical location of a subject (a system or a person), based on available information. This location capability is commonly performed by isolating a host system's IP address from a packet header, identifying the owner of the IP address range associated with the target system, discovering the owner's mailing address, and drilling down further -- with the objective of pinpointing the physical location of the target IP address (*What is Geolocation and How Does it Apply to Network Detection?*).

The suggested file security system encrypts the files using Rijndael Algorithm (AES), In order for the file to be stored in a more secured manner, the system uses two more security mechanisms (*AES: The Advanced Encryption Standard*). First, each file has a password associated with it, without which the file cannot be accessed. This password is defined by the user and stored in the database after being hashed using SHA-512 algorithm. Secondly, at the time the user uploads the file, the system records the user's current location and defines a trusted area, such that the file is accessible only within it. Therefore, when the user tries to access the file the system again captures the user's location and checks whether it is in the confinement of the trusted area. To provide additional security the location for describing the trusted area is also encrypted using the Rijndael Algorithm (AES).

Various existing techniques used for cloud storage have been discussed.

## Identity Based Authentication

In Cloud Computing, resources and services are distributed across numerous consumers. So there is a chance of various security risks. Therefore authentication of users as well as services is an important requirement for cloud security and trust. When SSL Authentication Protocol (SAP) was employed to cloud, it becomes very complex. As an alternative to SAP, proposed a new authentication protocol based on identity which is based on hierarchical model with corresponding signature and encryption schemes (Kahanwal, Dua & Singh, 2012).

## Efficient Third Party Auditing

A novel and homogeneous structure is introduced to provide security to different cloud types. To achieve data storage security, BLS (Boneh–Lynn–Shacham) algorithm is used to signing the data blocks before outsourcing data into cloud. BLS (Boneh–Lynn–Shacham) algorithm is efficient and safer than the former algorithms.

## Effective and Secure Storage Protocol

Current trend is users outsourcing data into service provider who have enough area for storage with lower storage cost. A secure and efficient storage protocol is proposed that guarantees the data storage confidentiality and integrity. This protocol is invented by using the construction of Elliptic curve cryptography and Sobol Sequence is used to confirm the data integrity arbitrarily. Cloud Server challenges a random set of blocks that generates probabilistic proof of integrity (Rajathi, & Saravanan, 2013).

## PROPOSED APPROACH

### User Login

1. Every user is assigned an ID and password at the time of registration.
2. This password is stored in the database after hashing using the hashing algorithm.
3. At the time of login, the users are prompted to enter their valid ID and password.
4. The entered password is hashed using the same algorithm and then matched with the password associated with the user in the database,
5. Once the user logs in, a session is established which allows the user to access the features of the system. i.e. unless one enters the valid credentials, one cannot access the system.

### File Upload and Storage Procedure

1. Once the user enters the system, he gets the option to upload a file.
2. The user can browse the system and select a text file to upload.
3. If the users tries to upload a file other than a text file, an error message is displayed prompting the user to select a text file.
4. Every file is associated with a password which is defined by the user at the time of uploading.

5. This password is hashed and stored in the database along with the path of the associated file.

6. The user also specifies a radius which is used while accessing the file to define a trusted area.

7. At the time of uploading the file, the user is given an option to specify the locations where the file can be accessed. The user can provide multiple access locations.

8. These locations are specified by giving the name of the locations on the map shown on the screen.

9. The system then obtains the co-ordinates of these locations specified by the user which are then encrypted and stored in the database.

## File Encryption Procedure

1. At the time of uploading, the text file is encrypted and stored at the server.

## File Download Procedure

1. Once the user logs in to the system, the user gets an option to download an already uploaded file.

2. The system displays the list of files uploaded by the user.

3. When the user selects a file for download, the system accesses the user's current coordinates.

4. The system decrypts the co-ordinates associated with the file and checks whether the current co-ordinates fall within the trusted area of the file using the radius given by the user at the time of file upload.

5. If the current co-ordinates fall within the trusted area, then the user is prompted for the password associated with the file, else the user is denied access to the file.

6. Only when both the co-ordinates as well the password are validated the user is granted access to the file.

## Hash Salt Algorithm

The basic hashing algorithm used is SHA-512. The message digest obtained from the algorithm is appended with the hash of a salt. The salt used is the user's login id for the user's login password and the id of the file for the file's password.

## Overview of SHA-512 (Data Protection for the Healthcare)

SHA-512 is a variant of SHA-256 which operates on eight 64-bit words. The message to be hashed is first:

1.  Padded with its length in such a way that the result is a multiple of 1024 bits long, and then;
2.  Parsed into 1024-bit message blocks M(1); M(2), .....,M(N). The message blocks are processed one at a time: Beginning with a fixed initial hash value H(0), sequentially compute:

$$H(i) = H(i-1) + CM(i) (H(i-1));$$

where C is the SHA-512 compression function and + means word-wise mod $2^{64}$ addition. H(N) is the hash of M.

## Encryption Algorithm

The algorithm used for encrypting the file and the coordinate values is the Rijndael Algorithm (AES). The key used in the algorithm is the message digest obtained after hashing the password entered by the user while accessing the file. The message digest is obtained using the ripemd128 algorithm.

## Overview of AES (Kahanwal, Dua & Singh, 2012)

AES is a block cipher with a block length of 128 bits. AES allows for three different key lengths: 128, 192, or 256 bits. With regard to using a key length other than 128 bits, the main thing that changes in AES is how you generate the key schedule from the key. Encryption consists of 10 rounds of processing for 128-bit keys, 12 rounds for 192-bit keys, and 14 rounds for 256-bit keys. Except for the last round in each case, all other rounds are identical. Each round of processing includes one single-byte based substitution step, a row-wise permutation step, a column-wise mixing step, and the addition of the round key. The order in which these four steps are executed is different for encryption and decryption.

## RESULTS

The basic UI design for the various functionalities mentioned above is given in Figures 1-8.

*Figure 1. Client Login Page: user has to enter valid user name and password to open account (http://php.net/docs.php)*

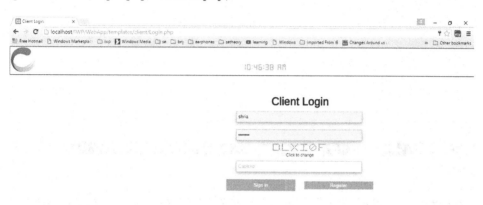

*Figure 2. Home Page*

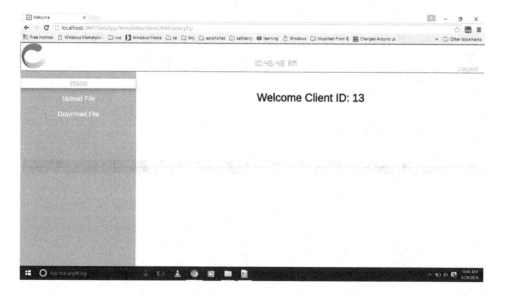

*Figure 3. File Upload Page: after successful login use has to upload file*

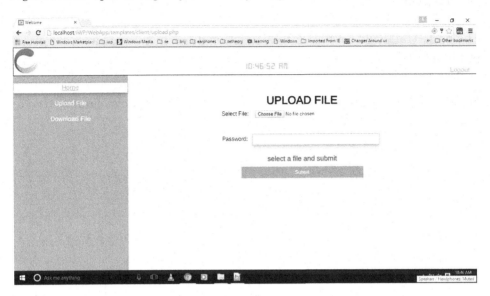

*Figure 4. File Upload: No File Selected. (http://www.iwar.org.uk/comsec/resources/cipher/sha256-384-512.pdf)*

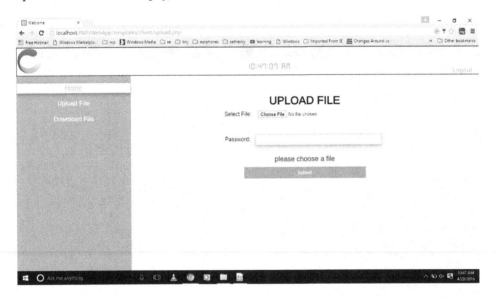

*Figure 5. File Upload: No Password Specified*

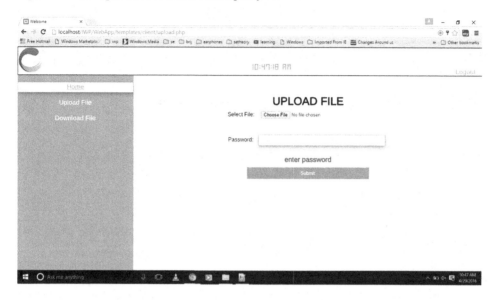

*Figure 6. File Upload: Internet Connectivity Error. (http://www.iwar.org.uk/comsec/ resources/cipher/sha256-384-512.pdf)*

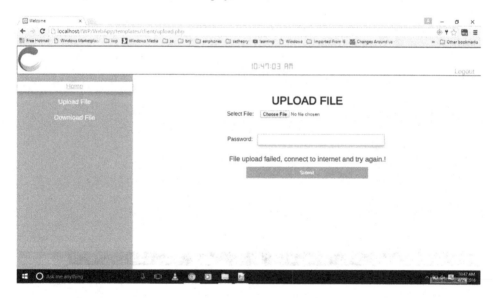

*Figure 7. File Upload Successful Message*

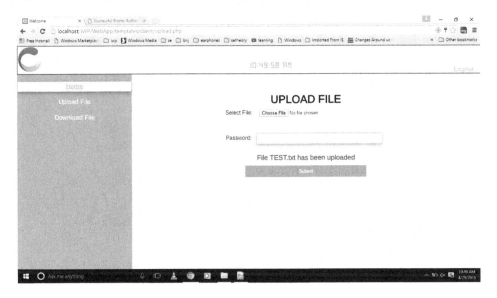

*Figure 8. File Download: Uploaded File List*

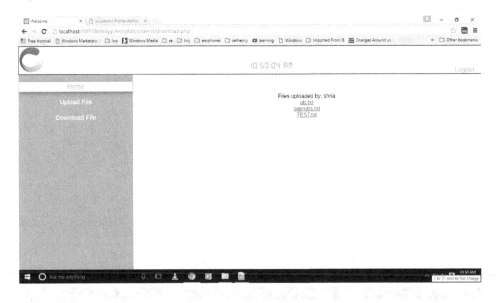

## CONCLUSION

The proposed system ensures the security of the file stored on the server by using a two factor verification method one of which is the password which is used to encrypt as well as access the file and the other utilizes the concept of a trusted area therefore ensuring that the file cannot be accessed by anyone unless they are at the right place and have the right credentials. Such kind of authentication process can be used to improve the file storage systems in hospitals and other services which record a user's personal and healthcare information and who want to store sensitive data and allow access to it only at certain specific locations.

## REFERENCES

AES. (n.d.). Retrieved from https://engineering.purdue.edu/kak/compsec / NewLectures/Lecture8.pdf

Data Protection for the Healthcare Industry. (n.d.). Retrieved from http:// www.safenet-inc.com/uploadedF iles/About_SafeNet/Resource_Library/ Resource_Items/White_PapersSFDC_Protected_EDP/SafeNet%20Data%20 Protection%20Healthcare%20White%20Paper.pdf

Kahanwal, Dua, & Singh. (2012). Java File Security System. *Global Journal of Computer Science and Technology Network and Web Security, 12*(10).

Rajathi, A., & Saravanan, N. (2013). A Survey on Secure Storage in Cloud Computing. *Indian Journal of Science and Technology, 6*(4).

Suhair, A. B., Golisano, T., Radziszowski, S. P., & Raj, R. K. (2012). Secure Access for Healthcare Data in the Cloud Using cipher text-Policy Attribute-Based Encryption. *Proc of International Conference on Data Engineering Workshop.*

What is Geolocation and How Does it Apply to Network Detection? (n.d.). Retrieved from https://www.sans.org/security-resources/idfaq/what-is-geolocation-and-how-does-it-apply-to-network-detection/1/28

# Chapter 8
# Clinical Data Analysis Using IoT Devices

**Govinda K.**
*VIT University, India*

## ABSTRACT

*The most recent couple of decades have seen a sharp rise in the number of elderly individuals. Furthermore, enquiry into this tells us that around 89% of the matured individuals are probably going to live autonomously. As the need be, giving a respectable personal satisfaction for matured individuals has turned into a genuine social test. Doctors need to have clear idea as to the health of these individuals, so they can use proper methodologies to cure them. Hence, IoT develops the idea of the internet and makes it more unavoidable. IoT permits consistent collaborations among various sorts of gadgets, for example, therapeutic sensors, observing cameras, home machines, and so on. This chapter proposes clinical data analysis using the internet of things.*

## INTRODUCTION

In the new era of communication and technology, the explosive growth of electronic devices, smart phones and tablets which can be communicated physically or wirelessly has become the fundamental tool of daily life. The next generation of connected world is Internet of Things (IoT) which connects devices, sensors, appliances, vehicles and other "things". The things or objects may include the radio-frequency identification (RFID) tag, mobile phones, sensors, actuators and much more. With the help of IoT, we connect

DOI: 10.4018/978-1-5225-5036-5.ch008

anything, access from anywhere and anytime, efficiently access any service and information about any object. The aim of IoT is to extend the benefits of Internet with remote control ability, data sharing, constant connectivity and so on. Using an embedded sensor which is always on and collecting data, all the devices would be tied to local and global networks.

Combining sensors and the microcontroller to get accurate measurement, and monitoring and analyzing the health status increase the power of IoT in healthcare. These can include blood pressure, heart rate, oxygen saturation in blood, levels of glucose and motion of body. For working effectively, smart sensors and microcontroller components have several capabilities: low power operation, integrated precision-analog capabilities and GUI's. To keep device footprint small and extend the life of battery to make the device usable, make the sensors possible to achieve high accuracy at low cost, improve the usability and read the information in a good manner. The end-to-end connectivity using sensors and other devices in healthcare. The server receives data of a person (who wearing several bio sensors) from the unit, then it feeds the sql data into its database and analyzes those data. Subsequently, based on the degree of abnormalities', it may interact with the family members of the person, local physician, or even emergency unit of a nearby healthcare center. Precisely, considering a person (not necessarily a patient) wearing several bio sensors on his body and the database receives a periodical updates from these sensors through IOT unit.

It allows the integration of intelligent, miniaturized low-power sensor nodes in, on or around human body to monitor body functions and the surrounding environment. It has great potential to revolutionize the future of healthcare technology. The proposed model provides platform for physical sensors, which are connected directly with patient's smartphone to obtain data at run time. This data is processed and stored in the MySql storage. The stored data can be accessed by practitioners and medical staff later on to observe and monitor patients' health and take decisions accordingly.

A barcode is an optical machine-readable representation of data relating to the object to which it is attached. Originally barcodes systematically represented data by varying the widths and spacing of parallel lines, and may be referred to as linear or one-dimensional (1D). Later they evolved into rectangles, dots, hexagons and other geometric patterns in two dimensions (2D). Although 2D systems use a variety of symbols, they are generally referred to as barcodes as well. Barcodes originally were scanned by special optical scanners called barcode readers. The Optical character recognition (OCR) and text to speech (TTS) an already practiced solution which detects barcode from the captured image and sent through smart phones. Two solutions are being proposed client framework for immediate solutions and the other hybrid cloud systems. The need of faster algorithms to give fast solutions in case of thousands of users. Classification and structuring among the pharmacy are yet to be done (GennaroTartarisco, Giovanni Baldus, Daniele Corda, RossellaRaso, AntoninoArnao, Marcello Ferro, Andrea Gaggioli, & Giovanni Pioggia, 2012).

A system for visually impaired to identify the products using smartphones with barcode and decode with text recognition on the users mobile device. A solution for blind to find the expiration date on the product package. Optical character recognition OCR algorithms are used to barcode detection to obtain the required information. System has produced a product barcode expiry date and has produced voice feedback on the products. The system is mainly for blind designed by blind experts and blind folded volunteers (Franca Delmastro, 2012).

An invisible barcode is generated in each medicine strip using steganography and barcode. The invisible barcode is generated in each strip and signed by a government authority. A cloud database is used that contain the list of the registered barcode of each medicine. By doing so we can avoid the expired and adulterated medicine (Altunkan, S.; Yasemin, A.; Aykac, I. & Akpinar, E., 2012).

In tradition QR scanning algorithm the pattern is recognized by a trial and error method in which it has to compare symbol with each the list of symbol and find the matching symbol. To overcome this a component labelling algorithm is used to compute a connected component and then find the inner most symbol of the connected component to find the pattern in the QR image (Jethjarurach, N. & Limpiyakorn, Y., 2014).

The importance of developing effective neuropharmaceuticals and the lack of efficacy of existing strategies for drug delivery to brain emphasize the need to develop new approaches to drug transport across the BBB[3]. Colloidal carrier system is a promising strategy for improving drug delivery to the brain[4]. These system includes micro spheres, liposomes, lipid micro spheres, polymer micelles, nanoparticles, solid lipid nano particles, niosomes, vector mediated BBB transport etc [5]. Nanotechnology is a break through technology expected to bring a revolutionary change in the field of life sciences including drug delivery, diagnostics, neutraceuticals and production of biomaterials[6].

Liposomes are the microscopic vesicles composed of one or more concentric lipid bilayers separated by water or aqueous buffer compartments with diameter ranging from 80 nm to 10 micron (Kailash, M.; Manokar, P. & Manokar, N. V., 2013).

In our present study, we have investigated the ability of surfactant modified liposomes to transport Evans blue dye without any damage to brain cortex. We have examined the suitable surfactant and their optimized molar concentration that modifies the liposomes to penetrate BBB towards delivering the entrapped molecule (Lin, S.-C. & Wang, P.-H., 2014).

A system to enable the blind users to find the date of manufacture and expiration date is based on a smart phone system that assist the blind user with the voice. The blind user is given a voice assistance to correctly locate the camera in smart phone to the bar code. Then the barcode decoding algorithm is used to decode the barcode. The resulting decoded information is then scanned by OCR app and converted into text, and delivered as a voice to blind people (Ohbuchi, E.; Hanaizumi, H. & Hock, L., 2004).

The expiry date detection of a product is very hard to find for a blind user. So a system processes that use a barcode decoder app and a text conversion app i.e OCR techniques to enable the blind user to know the expiry date by scanning through the barcode decoder app and then resulting is processed by a text recognition app to deliver it as an audio to the blind user (Ohsaga, A. & Kondoh, K., 2013).

## Literature Review

Health monitoring is an informal, non-statutory method of surveying your workforce for symptoms of ill health, including lower back pain. This type of occupational health management system can enable you, as an employer, to be aware of health problems and intervene to prevent problems being caused or made worse by work activities (X. Boyi, X. Li Da, C. Hongming, X. Cheng, H. Jingyuan, & B. Fenglin, 2014). Another important role of health monitoring is to give feedback into a system that reviews the current control methods in place (GennaroTartarisco, Giovanni Baldus, Daniele Corda, RossellaRaso, AntoninoArnao, Marcello Ferro, Andrea Gaggioli, & Giovanni Pioggia, 2012).

Automating design methodology (ADM) based on ontology is presented for smart rehabilitation system in IoT (F. Yuan Jie, Y. Yue Hong, X. Li Da, Z. Yan, & W. Fan, 2014). This architecture uses RFID, Wi-Fi, Bluetooth and cable network with Ethernet and TCP/IP. Some features of Artificial Intelligence are also applied to enhance the self-learning method of rehabilitation system. However, the limitation is this approach is that the records are entered manually while generation of rehabilitation strategy. Boyi et al (X. Boyi, X. Li Da, C. Hongming, X. Cheng, H. Jingyuan, and B. Fenglin, 2014) proposed a semantic data model to store and access the IoT data, and they also design a method called UDA-IoT to acquire and process the IoT ubiquity data. This architecture can also support the emergency medical services. The authors did not mention how will the data be obtained and is the model secure.

Sebestyen et al. (G. Sebestyen, A. Hangan, S. Oniga, & Z. Gal, 2014), implement and test an application called CardioNet, which is a distributed medical system linking different medical entities and systems like hospitals, emergency units, general practitioner cabinets, laboratories, personnel and patients. The implemented system is web based using ontology and can provide different services such as remote monitoring, online consultations, and hospital activity administration.

Boric-Lubecke et al (O. Boric-Lubecke, G. Xiaomeng, E. Yavari, M. Baboli, A. Singh, & V. M. Lubecke, 2014), discuss different applications of IoT in e-Healthcare. In particular, the authors focus on sleep studies and elderly care w.r.t remote monitoring applications. They explain the concept of Remote Sleep Monitoring and Elderly Monitoring in the context of IoT. They also discuss the privacy and security issues related to electronic medical data. Atzori et al (L. Atzori, A. Iera, & G. Morabito, 2010), conduct a survey on IoT and show different technologies and industrial standards which are already in use. The authors introduced and compared different visions of IoT paradigms, applications of IoT in medical like identification and authentication, tracking of patient flow or moment, data collection of patients, and sensing for diagnosing patent conditions.

It is a typical and a necessary provision available in the medical world. The main base for this is the clinical data management. IoT to helps us manage the clinical data. The Iot system used here requires a wireless networks to get data remotely, few embedded devices which we use on our day to day bases. The aim of clinical data management is to assure collection, integration and availability of data at appropriate quality and cost. As our system is present in our day today life it wouldn't be costly to upgrade the system to do another job that is to store that data for later analysis. The data will be available for the patient at any time and also for the hospitals to have an overview about the details of the patient. The other advantage of the system is that this information can be collected and used by scientist for research purpose and come up with an better solution [9]. The basic working of this system will be from the sensors taking the input and sending it to the smart phone which in turn send it to the server and the data is stored. With this the doctors can have live view over the patient's condition through the real time monitoring system which in turn helps the patients to get a better solution (Wan-Young Chung, Seung-Chul Lee, Sing-HuiToh, 2008); Strisland, F., Sintef,, Svagard, I., Seeberg, T.M., 2013).

In addition, there are specific regulations dealing with manual handling and whole body vibration in the workplace (Wan-Young Chung, Seung-Chul Lee, Sing-HuiToh, 2008). To ensure you are complying with your duties under these regulations you should refer to HSE (health system engineering) guidance, if manual h andling or whole body vibration are risks in your workplace (Strisland, F., Sintef,, Svagard, I., & Seeberg, T.M., 2013). Whole body vibration is particularly prevalent in those that drive industrial and parameters and the sampled parameters are wireless (BoyiXu, Li Da Xu,, HongmingCai, Cheng Xie, Jingyuan Hu, & Fenglin Bu, 2014).

RMMP-HI (Remote Monitoring & Management Platform of Healthcare Information) is presented by Wei et al (Z. Wei, W. Chaowei, & Y. Nakahira, 2011). The proposed platform is consisted of body sensors, a sensor network, wireless communication modules, home gateway or mobile phone/tablet and information storage. The authors analyze their platform with existing telemedicine services. Though different layers have been used in RMMP-Hi, but there is no information available on how will different layers communicates with each other and with the sensor, and what type of data storage is used.

## Proposed Method

The system is designed to monitor the status of the physical parameters. While monitoring there is data updating is happened, the system will send the data to the monitoring section. Then the data is visualized for better efficient decision making by the doctors. Hence making it easy and faster to take a decision into consideration.

It is mainly used for older people. The pressure sensor is used to monitor the patient's pressure status; the pulse sensor monitors the patient's heart beat and the temperature sensor monitors the temperature of the patient and sends to the microcontroller. If any value goes wrong means the it will be alert the surrounding people by blowing alarm. Also everything is transmitted via using bluetooth which can be viewed from any paired smartphone and the data will be stored in a pc.

Adding to this, an analysis graphs from the data from the Iot model into the My Sql Database, this data to create comparison graphs and the various inter relations of factors involving one's health this will enhance the doctors in better understanding of the patient and will help in taking the decisions faster than they actual time enhancing better chances of cure on a long term basis too.

For this purpose Tablueau isused, a data visualization which gives insight of data which can be connected in any format say a note or an excel or a word document, it groups the data and segregates itself according to the required points and then shows us all the metrics and we can then select the required metrics to compare and put in the various comparison graphs which has different types of graphs in it. So based on the need and requirement we can choose the graph, which serves our purpose and we can work accordingly.

*Figure 1. Block Diagram*

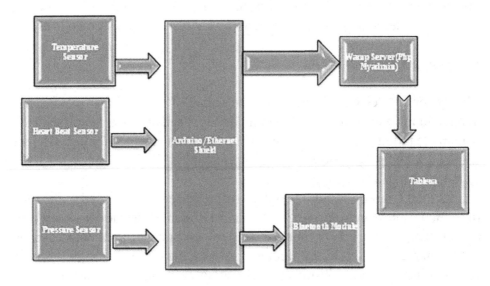

## ARDUINO UNO

Arduino/Genuino Uno is a microcontroller board based on the ATmega328P
. It has 14 digital input/output pins (of which 6 can be used as PWM outputs),
6 analog inputs, a 16 MHz quartz crystal, a USB connection, a power jack,
an ICSP header and a reset button. It contains everything needed to support
the microcontroller; simply connect it to a computer with a USB cable or
power it with a AC-to-DC adapter or battery to get started.

## Heart Beat Sensor

IR LED emits infrared radiation. This radiation illuminates the surface in
front of LED. Surface reflects the infrared light. Depending on reflectivity
of the surface, amount of light reflected varies. This reflected light is made
incident on reverse biased IR sensor. When photons are incident on reverse
biased junction of this diode, electron-hole pairs are generated, which results
in reverse leakage current. Amount of electron-hole pairs generated depends
on intensity of incident IR radiation. More intense radiation results in more
reverse leakage current. This current can be passed through a resistor so as

*Figure 2. Heart Beat Sensor*

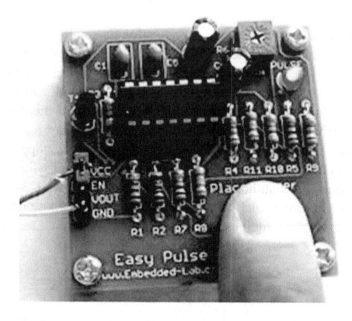

to get proportional voltage. Thus as intensity of incident rays varies, voltage across resistor will vary accordingly. This voltage can then be given to OPAMP based comparator. Output of the comparator can be read by uC. Alternatively, you can use on-chip ADC in microcontroller to measure this voltage and perform comparison in software.

## Temperature Sensor

Temperature is the most-measured process variable in industrial automation. Most commonly, a temperature sensor is used to convert temperature value to an electrical value. Temperature Sensors are the key to read temperatures correctly and to control temperature in industrials applications.

## Pressure Sensor

A pressure sensor measures pressure, typically of gases or liquids. Pressure is an expression of the force required to stop a fluid from expanding, and is usually stated in terms of force per unit area. A pressure sensor usually acts as a transducer; it generates a signal as a function of the pressure imposed. For the purposes of this article, such a signal is electrical.

## Bluetooth

Bluetooth is a de facto standard and specification for small-form factor, low-cost, short range radio links between mobile PCs, mobile phones and other portable devices. The technology allows users to form wireless connections between various communication devices, in order to transmit real-time voice and data communications. The Bluetooth radio is built into a small microchip and operates in the 2.4Ghz band, a globally available frequency band ensuring communication compatibility worldwide. It uses frequency hopping spread spectrum, which changes its signal 1600 times per second which helps to avoid interception by unauthorized parties. In addition software controls and identity coding built into each microchip ensure that only those units preset by their owners can communicate.

## Data Collection

Since before we analyze we need all the data into our data base we have the ethernet shield making the calls to the server by executing get request which enables the server to connect to the database and in this way the data obtained is saved into the database by using the add data php files which we have created in our www directory.

Now this data is classified already into various columns as we have already seen in our database structure. Now it is exported as an excel sheet with the same rows and columns.

The data collection from the arduino board is majorly by making Ethernet client connections with using the mac address and the ip address of the server. Then when the connection is established we can make calls to the server as

*Figure 3. Sample Data Set*

| Obs | BodyTemp | Gender | HeartRate | Pressure | BP | ECG | Glucose Levels | EEG(V) |
|-----|----------|--------|-----------|----------|----|-----|----------------|--------|
| 1 | 96.3 | Male | 70 | 93 | 65 | 575 | 126 | 4 |
| 2 | 96.7 | Male | 71 | 62 | 64 | 573 | 115 | 5 |
| 3 | 96.9 | Male | 74 | 81 | 65 | 572 | 100 | 3 |
| 4 | 97.0 | Male | 80 | 90 | 68 | 573 | 132 | 2 |
| 5 | 97.1 | Male | 73 | 72 | 72 | 575 | 100 | 3 |
| 6 | 97.1 | Male | 75 | 83 | 68 | 576 | 112 | 2 |
| 7 | 97.1 | Male | 82 | 96 | 65 | 578 | 117 | 2 |
| 8 | 97.2 | Male | 64 | 100 | 64 | 578 | 115 | 4 |
| 9 | 97.3 | Male | 69 | 71 | 63 | 579 | 112 | 5 |
| 10 | 97.4 | Male | 70 | 78 | 70 | 579 | 120 | 2 |
| 11 | 97.4 | Male | 68 | 99 | 65 | 577 | 118 | 4 |
| 12 | 97.4 | Male | 72 | 89 | 65 | 576 | 102 | 2 |
| 13 | 97.4 | Male | 78 | 83 | 60 | 576 | 124 | 4 |
| 14 | 97.5 | Male | 70 | 76 | 60 | 575 | 100 | 3 |
| 15 | 97.5 | Male | 75 | 84 | 65 | 572 | 99 | 5 |
| 16 | 97.6 | Male | 74 | 72 | 65 | 572 | 132 | 2 |
| 17 | 97.6 | Male | 69 | 91 | 60 | 570 | 120 | 4 |
| 18 | 97.6 | Male | 73 | 71 | 65 | 566 | 100 | 3 |
| 19 | 97.7 | Male | 77 | 76 | 65 | 566 | 113 | 2 |
| 20 | 97.8 | Male | 58 | 67 | 70 | 568 | 111 | 3 |
| 21 | 97.8 | Male | 73 | 70 | 75 | 568 | 115 | 3 |
| 22 | 97.8 | Male | 65 | 99 | 65 | 566 | 115 | 3 |
| 23 | 97.8 | Male | 74 | 93 | 64 | 564 | 132 | 2 |
| 24 | 97.9 | Male | 76 | 62 | 65 | 566 | 120 | 2 |
| 25 | 97.9 | Male | 72 | 81 | 68 | 566 | 100 | 4 |
| 26 | 98.0 | Male | 78 | 90 | 72 | 565 | 113 | 4 |
| 27 | 98.0 | Male | 71 | 72 | 68 | 564 | 111 | 5 |
| 28 | 98.0 | Male | 74 | 83 | 65 | 564 | 115 | 3 |
| 29 | 98.0 | Male | 67 | 96 | 64 | 563 | 115 | 2 |
| 30 | 98.0 | Male | 64 | 100 | 63 | 562 | 120 | 3 |
| 31 | 98.0 | Male | 78 | 71 | 70 | 559 | 112 | 2 |
| 32 | 98.1 | Male | 73 | 78 | 65 | 555 | 114 | 2 |

per our requirement, we also have a loop statement in our files which has the availability of looping the codes since we need multiple inputs in our database.

## Data Analysis

Now comes the major part of analyzing the data which can be done by using Tableau which is a data visualization tool helping to see the data as graphs, plot graphs, whisker graphs and others as per the requirement. The challenges we will be facing is which metrics to compare so that they will turn out to be useful for comparisons in our system.

Few Analysis Comparisons made are as follows.

In this the comparison between Blood Pressure and Heart Rate is made where a doctor based on this graph can evaluate how the patients heart rate varies with his blood pressure and by using this he can evaluate metrics like his sugar levels or if he is having heart problems or any blood low level issues.

The graph in Figure 5 shows that how the body temperature is affecting a patients Glucose levels, with this a doctor can evaluate a patients metabolism rate and accordingly the cure can be given pertaining to that body's functions.

In this we can see the variation of BP in males and females on a general basis, so hence we can also use it for general analysis or if pertaining to a specific region then that regions general trends can also be understood by the doctor.

*Figure 4. Blood Pressure vs. Heart Rate*

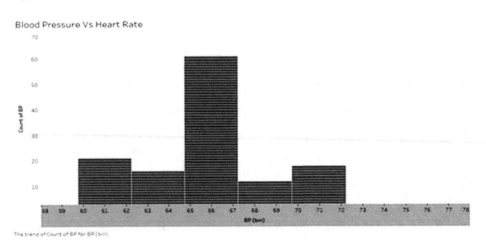

*Figure 5. Body Temperature vs. Glucose Levels*

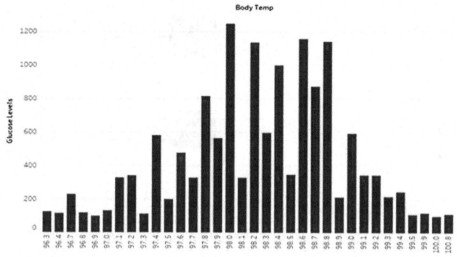

*Figure 6. Blood Pressure in Males and Females*

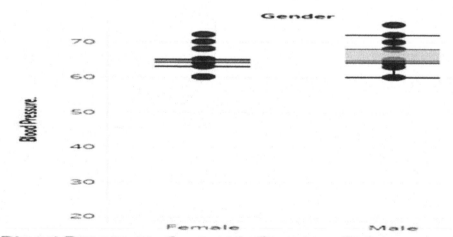

*Figure 7. ECG and Glucose Levels*

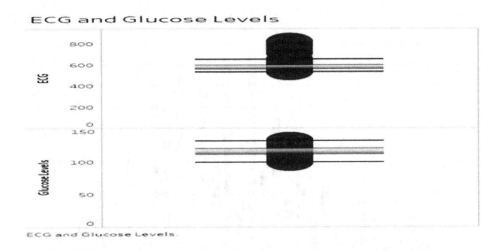

*Figure 8. ECG vs. Blood Pressure*

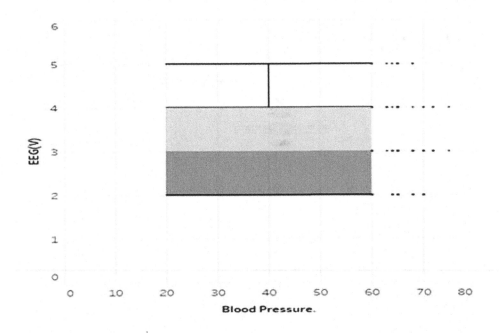

*Figure 9. Temperature vs. Pressure, Heart Rate and Glucose Levels*

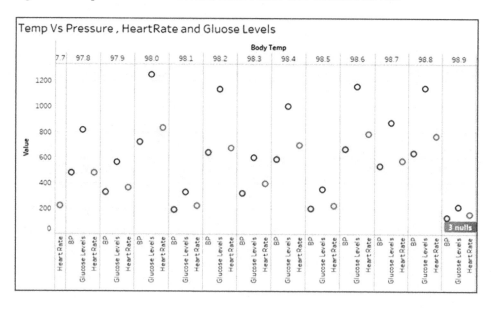

*Figure 10. Temperature vs. Blood Pressure*

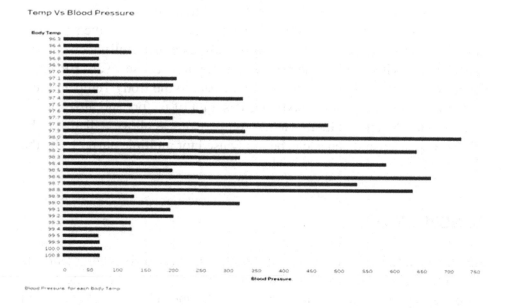

*Figure 11. Temperature vs. Glucose Levels and Pressure*

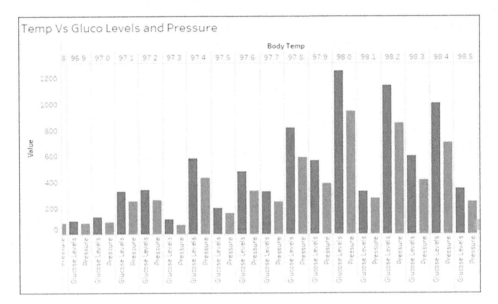

As we have seen ECG and Glucose levels and Blood Pressure in our body are interdependent so such comparisons also gives us insight as in how we evaluate the various patients functionality and their metabolism rates.

On a broader aspect when a doctor wants to refer to multiple metrics at the same time then he can refer to such analysis and create an overall understanding of the patient as it has many metrics like Heart rate, glucose levels, BP and at the same time all of them referring with respect to the Body Temperatures.

Temperature of a patients body decides a lot of factors and also a lot of other metrics depend on them. Hence comparisons as above will always be helpful to be used and hence can be easily used for multiple purposes by the doctor.

## CONCLUSION

It is a very intelligent technique to monitor the health. By the use of this system the health care sector can monitor, analyze, and provide the proper guidance required to advice the patients at all time. The physiological data can also be stored and used a record for the patient, whenever it is required in any later stages. This system also helps the professionals take care of their patients by monitoring the status online through their mobile devices.

The system is very power efficient. Only the smartphone or the tablet needs to be charged enough to do the test. It is easy to use, fast, accurate, high efficiency, and safe (without any danger of electric shocks). In contrast to other conventional medical equipment the system has the ability to save data for future reference. The system itself is a very simple but unique approach to the process of monitoring the health of a patient. It is integrated with sensors which help diagnose the patients in a very efficient manner. The data is also sent to the phone by enabling it through Bluetooth module. Implementing this system would help the hospitals monitor and diagnose patients in the best way possible using IOT processes. The reliability and validity of our system has been tested by using sample conditions and a set of data has been generated. The example tests show that the system can produce medical data that are similar to those produced by the existing medical equipment. So by using these analysis doctors can take smarter decisions for the treatment of the patients.

# REFERENCES

Altunkan, S., Yasemin, A., Aykac, I., & Akpinar, E. (2012). Turkish pharmaceuticals track amp; trace system. *7th International Symposium on in Health Informatics and Bioinformatics (HIBIT), 2012*, 24-30.

Atzori, Iera, & Morabito. (2010). The Internet of Things: A survey. *Computer Networks, 54*, 2787-2805.

Borgia, E. (2014). The Internet of Thigs vision: Key features, application and open issues. *Computer Communications, 54*, 131. doi:10.1016/j.comcom.2014.09.008

Boric-Lubecke, O., Xiaomeng, G., Yavari, E., Baboli, M., Singh, A., & Lubecke, V. M. (2014). E-healthcare: Remote monitoring, privacy, and security. *Microwave Symposium (IMS), 2014 IEEE MTT-S International*, 1-3. 10.1109/MWSYM.2014.6848602

Boyi, X., Li Da, X., Hongming, C., Cheng, X., Jingyuan, H., & Fenglin, B. (2014). Ubiquitous Data Accessing Method in IoT-Based Information System for Emergency Medical Services. *Industrial Informatics, IEEE Transactions on, 10*(2), 1578–1586. doi:10.1109/TII.2014.2306382

Boyi, X., Li Da, X., Hongming, C., Cheng, X., Jingyuan, H., & Fenglin, B. (2014). Ubiquitous Data Accessing Method in IoT-Based Information System for Emergency Medical Services. *Industrial Informatics, IEEE Transactions on, 10*(2), 1578–1586. doi:10.1109/TII.2014.2306382

Chung, Lee, & Toh. (2008). WSN based mobile u-healthcare system with ECG, blood pressure measurement function. *30th Annual International Conference of the IEEE, Engineering in Medicine and Biology Society*, 1533 – 1536.

Delmastro, F. (2012). Pervasive communications in healthcare. *Computer Communications, 35*(11), 1284–1295. doi:10.1016/j.comcom.2012.04.018

Jethjarurach, N., & Limpiyakorn, Y. (2014). Mobile Product Barcode Reader for Thai Blinds. *International Conference on Information Science and Applications (ICISA)*, 1-4. 10.1109/ICISA.2014.6847426

Kailash, M., Manokar, P., & Manokar, N. V. (2013). Scanmedic through e-governance. *7th International Conference on Intelligent Systems and Control (ISCO)*, 480-483.

Lin, S.-C., & Wang, P.-H. (2014). Design of a barcode identification system. *IEEE International Conference on Consumer Electronics - Taiwan (ICCE-TW)*, 237-238. 10.1109/ICCE-TW.2014.6904077

Ohbuchi, E., Hanaizumi, H., & Hock, L. (2004). Barcode readers using the camera device in mobile phones. *International Conference on Cyberworlds*, 260-265. 10.1109/CW.2004.23

Ohsaga, A., & Kondoh, K. (2013). Bedside medication safety management system using a PDA and RFID tags. *7th International Symposium on Medical Information and Communication Technology (ISMICT)*, 85-89. 10.1109/ISMICT.2013.6521705

Ong, S. K., Chai, D., & Rassau, A. (2011). A robust mobile business card reader using MMCC barcode. *IEEE Symposium on Computers Informatics (ISCI)*, 656-661. 10.1109/ISCI.2011.5958994

Parvu, O., Balan, A., & Homorogan, A. (2011). A case for online real-time barcode readers. *19th Telecommunications Forum (TELFOR)*, 1546-1549. 10.1109/TELFOR.2011.6143853

Peng, E., Peursum, P., & Li, L. (2012). Product Barcode and Expiry Date Detection for the Visually Impaired Using a Smartphone. *International Conference on Digital Image Computing Techniques and Applications (DICTA)*, 1-7. 10.1109/DICTA.2012.6411673

Sebestyen, G., Hangan, A., Oniga, S., & Gal, Z. (2014). eHealth solutions in the context of Internet of Things. *Automation, Quality and Testing, Robotics, 2014 IEEE International Conference*, 1-6. 10.1109/AQTR.2014.6857876

Strisland, F., Svagard, I., & Seeberg, T.M. (2013). ESUMS: A mobile system for continuous home monitoring of rehabilitation patient. *Proceedings of the 35th IEEE Annual International Conference on Engineering in Medicine and Biology Society*, 4670-4673.

Tartarisco, G., Baldus, G., Corda, D., Raso, R., Arnao, A., Ferro, M., ... Pioggia, G. (2012). Personal Health System architecture for stress monitoring and support to clinical decisions. *Computer Communications*, *35*(11), 1296–1305. doi:10.1016/j.comcom.2011.11.015

Touati, F., & Tabish, R. (2013). Towards u-health: An indoor 6LoWPAN based platform for real-time healthcare monitoring. *Proceedings of the IFIP International Conference on Wireless and Mobile Networking*, 1-4.

Wei, Z., Chaowei, W., & Nakahira, Y. (2011). Medical application on internet of things. *Communication Technology and Application (ICCTA 2011), IET International Conference on*, 660-665.

Weihua, W., Jiangong, L., Ling, W., & Wendong, Z. (2011). The internet of things for resident health information service platform research. *Communication Technology and Application (ICCTA 2011), IET International Conference on*, 631-635. 10.1049/cp.2011.0745

Xu, Xu, Cai, Xie, Hu, & Bu. (2014). Ubiquitous Data Accessing Method in IoT-Based Information System for Emergency Medical Services. *IEEE Transactions on Industrial Informatics*, *10*(2).

Yuan Jie, F., Yue Hong, Y., Li Da, X., Yan, Z., & Fan, W. (2014). IoT-Based Smart Rehabilitation System. *Industrial Informatics, IEEE Transactions on*, *10*(2), 1568–157. doi:10.1109/TII.2014.2302583

# Chapter 9
# Body Fitness Monitoring Using IoT Device

**Govinda K.**
*VIT University, India*

## ABSTRACT

*Recent technological advances in wireless communications and wireless sensor networks have enabled the design of intelligent, tiny, low-cost, and lightweight medical sensor nodes that can be placed on the human body strategically. The focus of this chapter is to implement the health monitoring system continuously without hospitalization using wearable sensors and create a wireless body area network (WBAN). Wearable sensors monitor the parameters of the human body like temperature, pressure, and heart beat by using sensors and providing real-time feedback to the user and medical staff and WBANs promise to revolutionize health monitoring. In this chapter, medical sensors are used to collect physiological data from patients and transmit it to the system which has details of an individual stored using Bluetooth/Wi-Fi with the help of Arduino and to medical server using Wi-Fi/3G communications.*

## INTRODUCTION

The health problem is rising along with increasing population in the today's world. In hospitals, continuous monitoring is needed for heart attack, after major/minor operation, temperature related illness, physical disorders. But the 24x7 monitoring of patients is difficult and leads to high cost. Wireless Sensor

DOI: 10.4018/978-1-5225-5036-5.ch009

Networks (WSNs) with intelligent sensor nodes are becoming significant enabling technology for wide range applications. Recent technology advances in integration and miniaturization of physical sensors, microprocessors, and radio interfaces on a single chip, have enabled a new generation of wireless sensor networks suitable for many applications. One of the most promising uses of WSNs is healthcare monitoring. In the medical field, sensor is used to collect the data about the person and send the information using wireless technology. This method reduces the health care cost of patients. A wireless sensor network consists of many nodes equipped with a sensing unit, memory, microcontroller (microprocessor), wireless communication interface and power source. WSNs can be deployed in an ad-hoc manner which make them robust, fault tolerance, and increase in spatial coverage. They can greatly be used to monitor and track conditions of patients in both cities and rural areas using an intranet or internet thereby reducing the stress and strain of healthcare providers, eliminate medical errors, reduce workload and increase efficiency of hospital staff, reduce long-term cost of healthcare services, and improve the comfort of the patients. Therefore, providing guaranteed, secured, and low transmission latency. The sensor nodes are being operated by batteries, their power consumption during transmission must be minimal for efficient and reliable data transmission between WBAN and personal server. Using sensor nodes with communication technologies such as mobile phones, General Packet Radio Service (GPRS), 3G, and the internet, the sensor network can keep patient, caregivers, and doctor informed while also establishing trends and detecting variations in health. The proposed system is to monitoring the patients continuously from remote areas using wearable sensors. This system consists of many sensors such as temperature, pressure, heart beat, and accelerometer. The data are collected by the sensors is calculated and analysed using microcontroller. Based on the predefined values it compares and displays the information about the patients.

## Literature Review

Physiological measures of interest in rehabilitation include heart rate, respiratory rate, blood pressure, blood oxygen saturation, and muscle activity. Parameters extracted from such measures can provide indicators of health status and have tremendous diagnostic value. Until recently, continuous monitoring of physiological parameters was possible only in the hospital setting. But today, with developments in the field of wearable technology, the possibility of accurate, continuous, real-time monitoring of physiological signals is a reality.

In recent years, physiological monitoring has benefited significantly from developments in the field of flexible circuits and the integration of sensing technology into wearable items (Barbaro, Caboni, Cosseddu, Mattana, & Bonfiglio, 2010). An ear-worn, flexible, low-power PPG sensor for heart rate monitoring was introduced by Patterson et al. (Patterson, McIlwraith, & Yang, 2009). The sensor is suited for long-term monitoring due to its location and unobtrusive design. Although systems of this type have shown promising results, additional work appears to be necessary to achieve motion artifact reduction (Yan, & Zhang, 2008, Wood, & Asadd, 2007). Proper attenuation of motion artifacts is essential to the deployment of wearable sensors. Some of the problems due to motion artifacts could be minimized by integrating sensors into tight fitting garments. A comparative analysis of different wearable systems for monitoring respiratory function was presented by Lanata et al. (2010). The analysis showed that piezoelectric pneumography performs better than spirometry. Nonetheless, further advances in signal processing techniques to mitigate motion artifacts are needed.

There has been a growing interest in the development of self-contained lab-on-a-chip systems. Such systems can revolutionize point-of-care medical testing and diagnosis by making testing and diagnosis fast, cheap and easily accessible. Wang et al. (2006) developed a system-on-chip (SOC), which integrates a pH and temperature sensor, for remote monitoring applications. Their SOC includes generic sensor interface, ADC, microcontroller, a data encoder and a frequency-shift keying RF transmitter. Similarly, Ahn et al. (2008) developed a low-cost disposable plastic lab-on-a-chip device for biochemical detection of parameters such as blood gas concentration and glucose. The biochip contains an integrated biosensor array for detecting multiple parameters and uses a passive microfluidic manipulation system instead of active microfluidic pumps.

Finally, applications in rehabilitation of remote monitoring systems relying on wearable sensors (Deshmukh, & Shilaskar, 2015) have largely relied upon inertial sensors for movement detection and tracking. Inertial sensors include accelerometers and gyroscopes. Often, magnetometers are used in conjunction with them to improve motion tracking. Today, movement sensors are inexpensive, small and require very little power, making them highly attractive for patient monitoring applications.

## Proposed Method

This device is used to measure the total steps a person walks with the device. The accelerometer used measures the force applied on it and by the force measured total steps can be calculated. The accelerometer detects force that is directed in the opposite direction from the acceleration vector. Most accelerometers will fall in two categories: digital and analog. Digital accelerometers will give you information using a serial protocol like I2C, SPI or USART, while analog accelerometers will output a voltage level within a predefined range that needs to get convert to a digital value using an ADC (analog to digital converter) module. Here the accelerometer gives a value to the processor which is the compared to a threshold value calibrated to steps we take. And according to the value the steps are counted. This device can further be used in different areas like to measure speed, calculate calories burned and all other things which need accelerometer.

*ADXL335* is a small, thin, low power, complete *3-axis accelero-meter* with signal conditioned voltage outputs. The product measures acceleration with a minimum full-scale range of $\pm3$ g. It can measure the static acceleration of gravity in tilt-sensing applications, as well as dynamic acceleration resulting from motion, shock, or vibration.

ADXL335 is 3v3 compatible device, it's powered by a 3.3v source and also generates 3.3v peak outputs. It has three outputs for each axis i.e. X, Y & Z. These are analog outputs and thus require an ADC in a micro-controller. Figure 1 shows arduino architecture which solves this problem. We will be using the analog functions of Arduino.

The Accelerometer module has 5 pins, namely:

1. GND-To be connected to Arduino's GND.
2. VCC-To be connected to Arduino's 5V.
3. X-To be connected to Analog Pin A5.
4. Y-To be connected to Analog Pin A4.
5. Z-To be connected to Analog Pin A3.

Most accelerometers will fall in two categories: digital and analog. Digital accelerometers will give you information using a serial protocol like I2C, SPI or USART, while analog accelerometers will output a voltage level within a predefined range that you have to convert to a digital value using an ADC

*Figure 1. Pin diagram of Arduino*

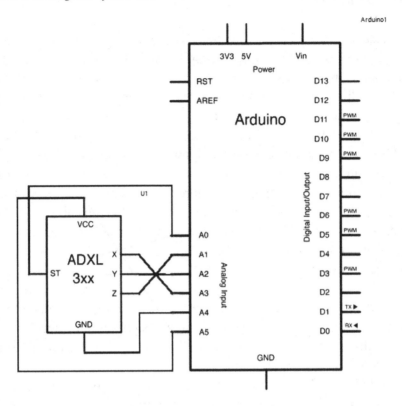

(analog to digital converter) module. Some microcontroller will have a built-in ADC modules some of them will need external components in order to perform the ADC conversions.

## About Accelerometer

An accelerometer is a device that measures proper acceleration. Accelerometers have multiple applications in industry and science. Accelerometers are used to detect and monitor vibration in rotating machinery. Highly sensitive accelerometers are components of inertial navigation systems for aircraft and missiles. Accelerometers are used in tablet computers and digital cameras so that images on screens are always displayed upright. Accelerometers are used in drones for flight stabilization. Figure 2 shows working process of proposed system. Coordinated accelerometers can be used to measure differences in

*Figure 2. Flow chart of proposed system*

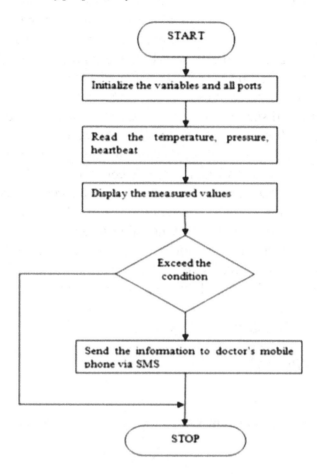

proper acceleration, particularly gravity, over their separation in space; i.e., gradient of the gravitational field. This gravity gradiometry is useful because absolute gravity is a weak effect and depends on local density of the Earth which is quite variable.

Single- and multi-axis models of accelerometer are available to detect magnitude and direction of the proper acceleration, as a vector quantity, and can be used to sense orientation (because direction of weight changes), coordinate acceleration, vibration, shock, and falling in a resistive medium (a case where the proper acceleration changes, since it starts at zero, then increases). Micromachined accelerometers are increasingly present in portable electronic devices and video game controllers, to detect the position of the device or provide for game input.

For better understanding think of accelerometers as a box in shape of a cube with a ball inside it. Imagine a ball with box as the outer-space far-far away from any cosmic bodies, or if such a place is hard to find imagine at least a space craft orbiting around the planet where everything is in weightless state. From the picture below you can see the assignment to each axis a pair of walls (the wall Y+ is removed so to look inside the box). Imagine that each wall is pressure sensitive. If suddenly the box is moved to the left (accelerate it with acceleration 1g = 9.8m/s^2), the ball will hit the wall X-. Then measure the pressure force that the ball applies to the wall and output a value of -1g on the X axis. Figure 3. shows x and y- axis accelerometer.

Please note that the accelerometer will detect a force that is directed in the opposite direction from the acceleration vector. This force is often called Inertial Force or Fictitious Force. One thing to learn from this is that an accelerometer measures acceleration indirectly through a force that is applied to one of its walls. This force can be caused by the acceleration. If the model is put on Earth the ball will fall on the Z- wall and will apply a force of 1g on the bottom wall.

Please notice the following relation:

$$R^2 = Rx^2 + Ry^2 + Rz^2 \qquad (1)$$

Let's move on by considering a simple example, suppose our 10bit ADC module gave us the following values for the three accelerometer channels (axes):

AdcRx = 586
AdcRy = 630
AdcRz = 561

*Figure 3. X and Y – AXIS Accelerometer*

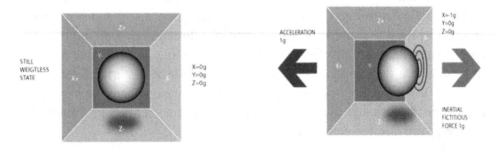

160

*Figure 4. Z – AXIS Accelerometer*

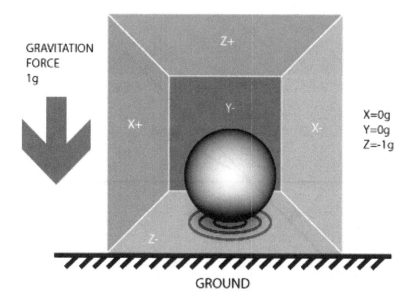

Each ADC module will have a reference voltage, let's assume for example it is 3.3V. To convert a 10bit adc value to voltage we use the following formula:

VoltsRx = AdcRx * Vref / 1023

A quick note here: that for 8bit ADC the last divider would be 255 = 2 ^ 8 -1, and for 12bit ADC last divider would be 4095 = 2^12 -1.

Applying this formula to all 3 channels we get:

VoltsRx = 586 * 3.3V / 1023 =~ 1.89V (we round to 2 decimal points)
VoltsRy = 630 * 3.3V / 1023 =~ 2.03V
VoltsRz = 561 * 3.3V / 1023 =~ 1.81V

Let's say 0g voltage level is VzeroG = 1.65V. To calculate the voltage shifts from zero-g voltage as follows:

DeltaVoltsRx = 1.89V - 1.65V = 0.24V
DeltaVoltsRy = 2.03V - 1.65V = 0.38V
DeltaVoltsRz = 1.81V - 1.65V = 0.16V

*Figure 5.*

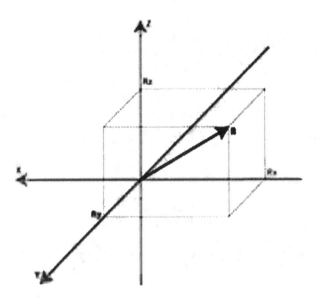

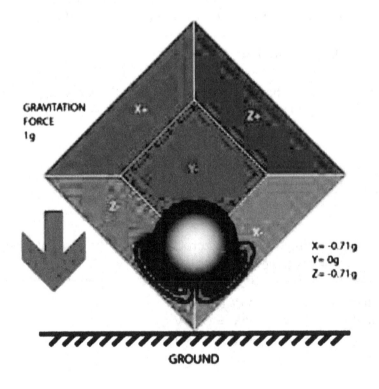

To do the final conversion apply the accelerometer sensitivity, usually expressed in mV/g. Let's say Sensitivity = 478.5mV/g = 0.4785V/g. Sensitivity values can be found in accelerometer specifications. To get the final force values expressed in g use the following formula:

Rx = DeltaVoltsRx / Sensitivity
Rx = 0.24V / 0.4785V/g =~ 0.5g
Ry = 0.38V / 0.4785V/g =~ 0.79g
Rz = 0.16V / 0.4785V/g =~ 0.33g
Rx = (AdcRx * Vref / 1023 - VzeroG) / Sensitivity (Equation 2)
Ry = (AdcRy * Vref / 1023 - VzeroG) / Sensitivity
Rz = (AdcRz * Vref / 1023 - VzeroG) / Sensitivity.

Some additional notations

R = SQRT(Rx^2 + Ry^2 + Rz^2)

*Figure 6.*

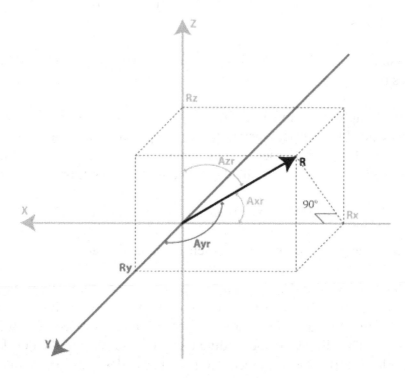

## Calorie Calculation

Casual Walking - 2 mph

**Step 1:** Multiply the weight by 0.57 to calculate how many calories you burn in 1 mile of casual walking. This factor is based on a formula that calculates calories burned when a person walks at a casual pace of 2 mph. For example, if someone weighs 121 lbs. the calculation would look like this:

Calories burned per mile = 0.57 x 121 lbs. = 68.97 calories per mile.

**Step 2:** Walk casually for exactly 1 mile while wearing your pedometer. Record the number of steps it took to walk that mile. For example, it may have taken 2,200 steps.

**Step 3:** Divide the number of calories you burn per mile by the number of steps it takes to walk a mile. The result is a unique-to conversion factor and can be used to calculate how many calories are burnt from the number of steps taken. For example, the calculation would look like this for a person who burns 68.97 calories per mile and walks a mile in 2,200 steps:

Conversion factor = 68.97 calories per mile / 2,200 steps per mile = 0.03135 calories per step

**Step 4:** Multiply the conversion factor by the number of steps you take, as indicated by your pedometer, during any given walk to figure out how many calories are burned. For example, if the person from the example walked 7,000 steps, the calculation would look like this:

Calories burned = 7,000 steps x 0.03135 calories per step = 219 calories

Some of the applications of wireless sensors in healthcare:

1. **Heart Diseases:** Cardiovascular disease refers to various medical conditions that affect the heart and blood vessels. The conditions include heart attack, heart failure, stroke, coronary artery disease (Rosamond, 2007). This disease is the leading cause of mortality in the developed world. A WBAN is a key technology that provides real-time monitoring

of cardiovascular patients by continuously sense, process, and transmit physiological data from central control unit to the medical server through personal server, which the physician can make use of the information to treat the patients (Shany, Redmond, Narayanan, & Lovell, 2012; Suryadevara, & Mukhopadhyay, 2012).

2. **Asthma:** A WBAN can help millions of patients who are suffering from asthma in the world, by monitoring allergic agents in the air and providing real-time feed-back to the physician and/or to the patient himself. A portable Global Positioning System (GPS) device was developed that continuously consults a remote server by sensing user's reports to decide whether current ambient air quality will threaten user's health.

3. **Cancer Detection:** Cancer is now one of the biggest threats to the human life. A WBAN with a set of miniaturized sensors can be used to differentiate between different types of cells and identifying cancerous cells, enabling physicians to diagnose tumors without biopsy.

4. **Diabetes:** Complications that occurs as a result of diabetes: amputations, blindness, kidney disease, stroke, high blood pressure, heart disease Treatment includes blood pressure control, exercise, insulin injections (Zhao, Davidson, Bain, Li, Wang, & Lin, 2005). A WBAN can be used in a more effective way to treat diabetes, by providing a more consistent, less invasive and accurate method for monitoring glucose levels in the body.

5. **Artificial Retina:** Optoelectronic Retina Prosthesis (ORP) chips can be implanted into the back of human eye, which assist blinds and/or patients with low vision to see normally.

## System Architecture

This section describes the system architecture in Figure 7 of the proposed wearable sensors for remote healthcare monitoring system (Wang, Yang, Huang, Zhang, Yu, Nie, & Cumming, 2010: Khemapech, 2005; She, Lu, Jantsch, Zheng, & Zhou, 2007). The system is composed of three tiers namely:

1. Wireless Body Area Network (WBAN) (Jovanov, Milenkovic, Otto, & De Groen, 2005);
2. Personal Server (Milenković, Otto, & Jovanov, 2006);
3. Medical Server for Healthcare Monitoring (MSHM) (Bonato, 2005; Lo, & Yang, 2005).

*Figure 7. System Architecture*

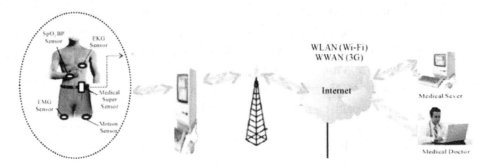

# RESULTS

Successful and accurate calculation of number of steps, distance covered and amount of energy burned by an individual.

# CONCLUSION

With *ADXL335* which is a *3-axis accelerometer.* It can calculate number of steps holding the device in hand, distance covered and also the amount of fat burned during walking. With this device on further advancement the size of hardware can be decreased and can be used in different devices which need acceleration. Application can be in robotic devices, fitness band, speedometer and many more.

# REFERENCES

Barbaro, M., Caboni, A., Cosseddu, P., Mattana, G., & Bonfiglio, A. (2010). Active devices based on organic semiconductors for wearable applications. *IEEE Transactions on Information Technology in Biomedicine, 14*(3), 758–766. doi:10.1109/TITB.2010.2044798 PMID:20371414

Bonato, P. (2005). Advances in wearable technology and applications in physical medicine and rehabilitation. *Journal of Neuroengineering and Rehabilitation, 2*(1), 2. doi:10.1186/1743-0003-2-2 PMID:15733322

Deshmukh, S. D., & Shilaskar, S. N. (2015, January). Wearable sensors and patient monitoring system: A Review. In *Pervasive Computing (ICPC), 2015 International Conference on* (pp. 1-3). IEEE. 10.1109/PERVASIVE.2015.7086982

Dudde, R., Vering, T., Piechotta, G., & Hintsche, R. (2006). Computer-aided continuous drug infusion: Setup and test of a mobile closed-loop system for the continuous automated infusion of insulin. *IEEE Transactions on Information Technology in Biomedicine, 10*(2), 395–402. doi:10.1109/TITB.2006.864477 PMID:16617628

Jovanov, E., Milenkovic, A., Otto, C., & De Groen, P. C. (2005). A wireless body area network of intelligent motion sensors for computer assisted physical rehabilitation. *Journal of Neuroengineering and Rehabilitation, 2*(1), 6. doi:10.1186/1743-0003-2-6 PMID:15740621

Khemapech. (2005). *A Survey of Wireless Sensor Net-works Technology. In 6th Annual Postgraduate Symposium on the Convergence of Telecommunications, Networking and Broadcasting.* Liverpool, UK: Liverpool John Moores University.

Lanatà, A., Scilingo, E. P., Nardini, E., Loriga, G., Paradiso, R., & De-Rossi, D. (2010). Comparative evaluation of susceptibility to motion artifact in different wearable systems for monitoring respiratory rate. *IEEE Transactions on Information Technology in Biomedicine, 14*(2), 378–386. doi:10.1109/TITB.2009.2037614 PMID:20007035

Lo, B., & Yang, G. Z. (2005, April). Key technical challenges and current implementations of body sensor networks. *Proc. 2nd International Workshop on Body Sensor Networks (BSN 2005).*

Milenković, A., Otto, C., & Jovanov, E. (2006). Wireless sensor networks for personal health monitoring: Issues and an implementation. *Computer Communications, 29*(13), 2521–2533. doi:10.1016/j.comcom.2006.02.011

Morris, D., Schazmann, B., Wu, Y., Coyle, S., Brady, S., Fay, C., . . . Diamond, D. (2008, August). Wearable technology for bio-chemical analysis of body fluids during exercise. In *Engineering in Medicine and Biology Society, 2008. EMBS 2008. 30th Annual International Conference of the IEEE* (pp. 5741-5744). IEEE. 10.1109/IEMBS.2008.4650518

Patterson, J. A., McIlwraith, D. C., & Yang, G. Z. (2009, June). A flexible, low noise reflective PPG sensor platform for ear-worn heart rate monitoring. In *Wearable and Implantable Body Sensor Networks, 2009. BSN 2009. Sixth International Workshop on* (pp. 286-291). IEEE. 10.1109/BSN.2009.16

Rosamond, W., Flegal, K., Friday, G., Furie, K., Go, A., Greenlund, K., ... Hong, Y. (2007). American Heart Association Statistics Committee and Stroke Statistics Subcommittee. Heart disease and stroke statistics-2007 update: A report from the American heart association statistics committee and stroke statistics subcommittee. *Circulation, 115*(5), e69–e171. doi:10.1161/CIRCULATIONAHA.106.179918 PMID:17194875

Shany, T., Redmond, S. J., Narayanan, M. R., & Lovell, N. H. (2012). Sensors-based wearable systems for monitoring of human movement and falls. *IEEE Sensors Journal, 12*(3), 658–670. doi:10.1109/JSEN.2011.2146246

She, H., Lu, Z., Jantsch, A., Zheng, L. R., & Zhou, D. (2007, August). A network-based system architecture for remote medical applications. In *Network Research Workshop (Vol. 27)*. Academic Press.

Suryadevara, N. K., & Mukhopadhyay, S. C. (2012). Wireless sensor network based home monitoring system for wellness determination of elderly. *IEEE Sensors Journal, 12*(6), 1965–1972. doi:10.1109/JSEN.2011.2182341

Wang, L., Yang, G. Z., Huang, J., Zhang, J., Yu, L., Nie, Z., & Cumming, D. R. S. (2010). A wireless biomedical signal interface system-on-chip for body sensor networks. *IEEE Transactions on Biomedical Circuits and Systems, 4*(2), 112–117. doi:10.1109/TBCAS.2009.2038228 PMID:23853318

Wood, L. B., & Asada, H. H. (2007, August). Low variance adaptive filter for cancelling motion artifact in wearable photoplethysmogram sensor signals. In *Engineering in Medicine and Biology Society, 2007. EMBS 2007. 29th Annual International Conference of the IEEE* (pp. 652-655). IEEE. 10.1109/IEMBS.2007.4352374

Yan, Y. S., & Zhang, Y. T. (2008). An efficient motion-resistant method for wearable pulse oximeter. *IEEE Transactions on Information Technology in Biomedicine, 12*(3), 399–405. doi:10.1109/TITB.2007.902173 PMID:18693507

Zhao, Y. J., Davidson, A., Bain, J., Li, S. Q., Wang, Q., & Lin, Q. (2005, June). A MEMS viscometric glucose monitoring device. In *Solid-State Sensors, Actuators and Microsystems, 2005. Digest of Technical Papers. TRANSDUCERS'05. The 13th International Conference on* (Vol. 2, pp. 1816-1819). IEEE. 10.1109/SENSOR.2005.1497447

# Chapter 10
# Reading Assistance for Visually Impaired People Using TTL Serial Camera With Voice

**Sruthi M.**
*VIT University, India*

**Rajasekaran R.**
*VIT University, India*

## ABSTRACT

*Internet of things is where all the things are connected to the internet and communicate with each other. There are many applications of the IoT in various fields such as healthcare, agriculture, industries, and logistics, and even for empowering people with disabilities. There are many previous work for the blind people using IoT in finding the obstacles many navigation applications have been developed. In this chapter, a system is proposed to assist blind people in reading books. This method is based on capturing the text book pages as an image and processing them into text with speech as an output.*

## INTRODUCTION

The recent technologics have transformed the lifestyle of each person with increased comfort and extended the lifetime of each person. IOT is an emerging technology in which each thing is connected through an internet and makes communication in an automated environment. This can also apply for the providing services for the handicapped people. The challenges of the

DOI: 10.4018/978-1-5225-5036-5.ch010

blind people are in finding the obstacle in front of them, reading the books because not all the books are available in a braille method. The difficulty in braille method is printed the braille book and the maintenance of the braille book as all the holes printed in the braille book tend to fade away soon due to constant usage and storing method of the braille book. To avoid this system is proposed in which the text is captured as an image in a JPEG format. The captured image is then transmitted to the smart phone through WIFI. The image is then converted into the text using OCR app in a Smartphone. Text is converted into audio for visually impaired people; the converted text is stored in cloud for future use.

The paper is organized as follows:

The second part consisted of the previous work in assistance to the visually impaired people. The third part consists of design of reading assistance for the visually impaired people using TTL series cameras with the voice as an output. The design components are explained in a fourth part follows by conclusion as the fifth part.

## BACKGROUND

A service named Pharos is provided for the blind people to provide services such as to identify their current location, to find a correct route to their destination, to track their movement in the current location and send a message to other people about a meeting. These services are assisted by a GP and a gsm combined mobile phone that sends an SMS to a server. Then the admin at the server will provide the services by giving a recorded voice call or the request seeks by blind people are sent to a call center. From call center the information is provided as voice call to blind people (Marsh, May, & Saarelainen, 2000). To aid the elderly and handicapped people in their walking activities and to avoid from falling down a cane robot is designed that use a force sensor to determine the intention on their walking, a tilt angle sensor to control and to prevent from falling and it has three Omni wheel (Wakita, Huang, Di, Sekiyama, & Fukuda, 2013). A force blinker 2 a navigation tool for visually impaired people that uses a repulsive magnet to stop the false object detection to create by noise that increases the recognition of object in front of the blind people [Ando, T etal, 2012].Open source software named Nanodesktop is used to aid the visually impaired people for handling the computer with a voice assistance. Thus it is economical too since it is an open source software SDK which is free of cost to users (Battaglia, & Iannizzotto, 2012). An IOT architecture for disabled people is proposed a system that has a TCP/IP stack layers and each layers are explained their functionality such as device identification, and how the data are transmitted to the destination in a network, and how the interface are used for the various applications are discussed (Hussain, 2017). For elderly people and the disabled people an automated home control is proposed in which the user the places the android or an IOS phone camera towards an object then a virtual object menu by an wikitude SDK which pop's out in their phone and they can control the object with that and it also assisted using a voice control. In the background a ARCHServ is a server running backend to control the device (Tang, Ang, Amirul, Yusoff, Tng, Alyas,... & Folianto, 2015). The blind user wears an RGB-D sensor that can be worn at the waist and a head mounted camera through which the user can recognize the object before them and the crowd before them and any social gatherings through tweeting, and through Wi-Fi connection, communication they can get access to the geographical information, social media and the user is provided an audio speaker near the ear to deliver the audio as an assistant (Joseph, Xiao, Chawda, Narang, & Janarthanam, 2014). An IOT infrastructure for the visually impaired is proposed were the all things and places are tagged using RFID, QR code or NFC and assigned a unique code called ucode of 128 bits. A web server that contains a list of ucode and their corresponding information related to that thing or place is stored the user can get access to it by Wi-Fi or mobile communication through a sassy web api. Then the navigation information is provided to visually impaired people through a webapi called SaSYS. The visually impaired user gets the information needed by each gesture, i.e. for each gesture a service is provided. So based on the service needed for the visually impaired people the gesture differs (Kim, Bessho, Koshizuka, & Sakamura, 2014).

## FUNCTION OF MAJOR COMPONENTS

### TTL Serial Camera

The TTL serial does two functions: i) takes a video of NTSC video; ii) takes a snapshot of the video when a motion is detected. The reason to use the

TTL serial camera is it has features like auto brightness, auto balance and auto white balance which could be more helpful for the blind people. It has an in building JPEG compression engine to compress the picture in a JPEG format. It is low cost, consumes low power with high resolution picture. It also can detect the motion, which is used in this system by whenever there is a motion, i.e. When the user opens a book or turns a page, then it captures then it triggers to capture the page as a picture.

## Arduino Due

The reason to use an Arduino due than the Arduino UNO is in order to process the high resolution image it has a SRAM of 96 KB and flash memory of 512 KB. So Arduino due is preferred to capture a high resolution image.

## CC3000 WIFI CHIP

This chip contains a built in wireless network processor, IEEE 802.11b/g that is used to simplify the internet connectivity. It has an implanted IPV4 TCP/IP stacks. TX power +18.0 dBm at 11 Mbps, CCK RX sensitivity 88 dBm, 8% PER, 11 Mbps.

## OCR Technology

There are two different ways the OCR retrieves the text i) First the structure of the document image or a paper image is analyzed and then divide each letter, compare each letter image with the store copy of the letter and guess the letter. Another way is by feature detection; it detects the features such as angle, curves etc. and detects the letter. There are many OCR apps being available for Android, IOS, windows phone that can be useful for the detection of text from the images.

*Figure 1. A Reading Assistance for visually impaired people using TTL serial cameras and OCR technique with voice assistance*

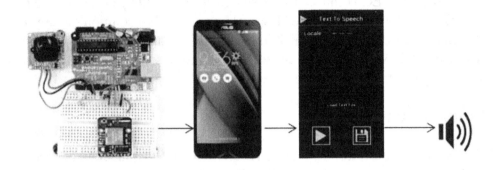

## PROPOSED SYSTEM

## TTL Serial Camera Connected to an Arduino Board With ACC300 WIFI Chip

The proposed system is meant for visually impaired people to help them with reading book's. the working of the system is it consist of a camera, to capture a page as an image. TTL serial camera is used to capture the image. Using a TTL serial camera is, it has an inbuilt feature's such as auto brightness, auto white adjustment which is important for the image clarity. The other reason for using a TTL serial camera is it can detect the motion and it captures the image, using this we capture a image. i.e when the user turn's the book the motion is detected and captures the page's as an image. Now the captured image consisted of text. The text has to retrieve from the image. The captured image is stored in the Arduino due processor. the capture image has to be processed to retrieve the text, so we use an CC3000 wifi to transmit the image from the Arduino due processor to the user's mobile. The transmitted image that contains text is then processed by an OCR app to retrieve the text from the image. Now the image is processed by an OCR app to convert the image to text. The OCR app can convert the image to text only when the image is clear. We use TTL serial camera as said before that has an auto brightness and auto white adjustment which will be helpful for the blind user's. Then the image is selected which has to be converted to text and the resulting text is delivered as an audio or speech. Since the user of this system is a visually impaired people the selection of the image and the other option's such as play as speech is done with the help of the google Talkback. The google Talkback tells the user what they have done with an audio. Then the retrieved text is then delivered as an audio or it can be shared to their friend's through communication app or can be saved in google drive or Dropbox for future use. An active WIFI connection is needed for the working of the proposed system as we have to transform the image, for working an OCR app to deliver it as a speech, for sharing purpose and for storing for future. The OCR app is able to support major languages and it also has an option for to download a language pack that is not supported or didn't have a language software pack in it by default. So this can used be all user all over the world.

*Figure 2. The app showing the image to select an image*

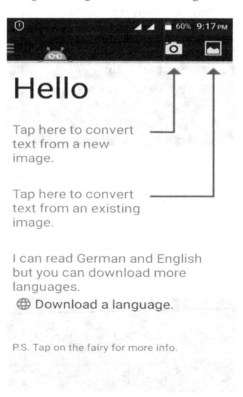

*Figure 3. The list of image the from which we have select the image*

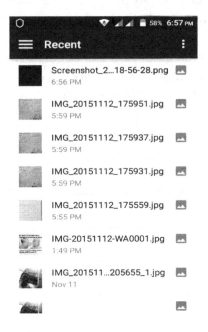

*Figure 4. The image is select and convert as a text*

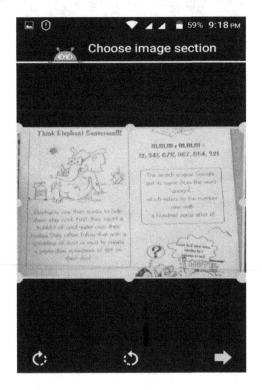

*Figure 5. Recognizing the text. from the image*

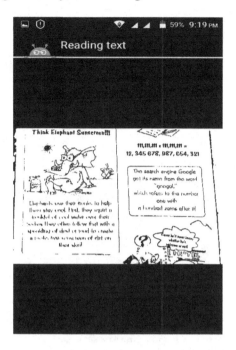

*Figure 6. Converting the recognized text from image to a text*

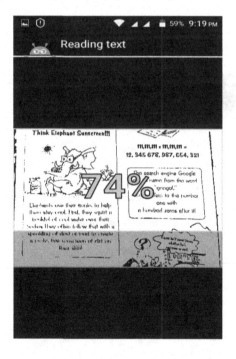

*Figure 7. The retrieved text. from the image*

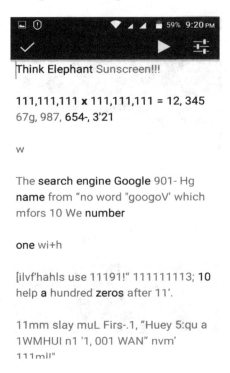

*Figure 8. Option to show the facility to read it as a text and to share the text in Dropbox or google drive*

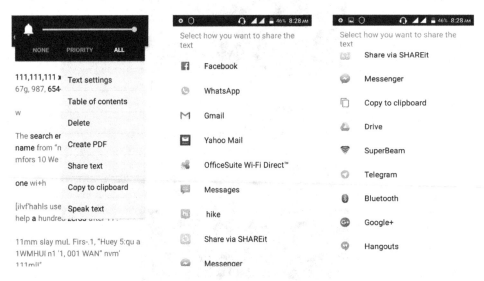

## EXPERIMENTAL ANALYSIS

An image which contains both the picture and text is captured. Now that image is used to by the user to convert it a text. The following screenshots shows how the image is chosen by the user with the help of Google Talkback and chooses the image, the image is processed, converted in to the text, the app provides an option of speaking the retrieved text and that also has an option to share the retrieved text with the others using many communication app, storing the text in Google Drive, Dropbox (see Figures 2-8).

## CONCLUSION

The reading aid for the visually impaired people is a better way for the blind people to find their own books and can read it independently. The TTL serial camera is a low cost, energy efficiency that can operate in 5v. The Arduino due microcontroller used is to store a snapshot of high resolution and has high processing speed. There are many OCR apps available in the play store for free of cost. And the blind people can operate it on their own using voice command. This can also be used to find the current place where they are. And in the future this system can be further developed by storing the text retrieved from the image in cloud for future use. This system can also be extended for security purpose of the blind people as the TTL serial camera is able to record the video.

## REFERENCES

Ando, T., Tsukahara, R., Seki, M., & Fujie, M. G. (2012). A haptic interface "Force blinker 2" for navigation of the visually impaired. *IEEE Transactions on Industrial Electronics, 59*(11), 4112–4119. doi:10.1109/TIE.2011.2173894

Battaglia, F., & Iannizzotto, G. (2012). An open architecture to develop a handheld device for helping visually impaired people. *IEEE Transactions on Consumer Electronics, 58*(3), 1086–1093. doi:10.1109/TCE.2012.6311360

Hussain, M. I. (2017). Internet of Things: challenges and research opportunities. *CSI Transactions on ICT, 5*(1), 87-95.

Joseph, S. L., Xiao, J., Chawda, B., Narang, K., & Janarthanam, P. (2014, June). A blind user-centered navigation system with crowdsourced situation awareness. In *Cyber Technology in Automation, Control, and Intelligent Systems (CYBER), 2014 IEEE 4th Annual International Conference on* (pp. 186-191). IEEE. 10.1109/CYBER.2014.6917458

Kim, J. E., Bessho, M., Koshizuka, N., & Sakamura, K. (2014, December). Mobile applications for assisting mobility for the visually impaired using IoT infrastructure. In *TRON Symposium (TRONSHOW)*, 2014 (pp. 1-6). IEEE.

Marsh, A., May, M., & Saarelainen, M. (2000). Pharos: coupling GSM and GPS-TALK technologies to provide orientation, navigation and location-based services for the blind. In *Information Technology Applications in Biomedicine, 2000. Proceedings. 2000 IEEE EMBS International Conference on* (pp. 38-43). IEEE. 10.1109/ITAB.2000.892345

Tang, L. Z. W., Ang, K. S., Amirul, M., Yusoff, M. B. M., Tng, C. K., Alyas, M. D. B. M., . . . Folianto, F. (2015, April). Augmented reality control home (ARCH) for disabled and elderlies. In *Intelligent Sensors, Sensor Networks and Information Processing (ISSNIP), 2015 IEEE Tenth International Conference on* (pp. 1-2). IEEE.

Wakita, K., Huang, J., Di, P., Sekiyama, K., & Fukuda, T. (2013). Human-walking-intention-based motion control of an omnidirectional-type cane robot. *IEEE/ASME Transactions on Mechatronics, 18*(1), 285–296. doi:10.1109/TMECH.2011.2169980

# Related References

To continue our tradition of advancing information science and technology research, we have compiled a list of recommended IGI Global readings. These references will provide additional information and guidance to further enrich your knowledge and assist you with your own research and future publications.

Aas, I. H. (2013). Improving patient safety with telemedicine: Exploring organizational factors. In A. Moumtzoglou & A. Kastania (Eds.), *E-health technologies and improving patient safety: Exploring organizational factors* (pp. 56–70). Hershey, PA: IGI Global. doi:10.4018/978-1-4666-2657-7.ch004

Aboelfotoh, M. H., Martin, P., & Hassanein, H. (2013). Ubiquitous multimedia data access in electronic health care systems. In D. Tjondronegoro (Ed.), *Tools for mobile multimedia programming and development* (pp. 191–227). Hershey, PA: IGI Global. doi:10.4018/978-1-4666-4054-2.ch011

Abreu, J. F., Almeida, P., & Silva, T. (2013). iNeighbour TV: A social TV application to promote wellness of senior citizens. In R. Martinho, R. Rijo, M. Cruz-Cunha, & J. Varajão (Eds.), Information systems and technologies for enhancing health and social care (pp. 1-19). Hershey, PA: IGI Global. doi:10.4018/978-1-4666-3667-5.ch001

Aceti, V., & Luppicini, R. (2013). Exploring the effect of mhealth technologies on communication and information sharing in a pediatric critical care unit: A case study. In J. Tan (Ed.), *Healthcare information technology innovation and sustainability: Frontiers and adoption* (pp. 88–108). Hershey, PA: IGI Global. doi:10.4018/978-1-4666-2797-0.ch006

Adami, I., Antona, M., & Stephanidis, C. (2014). Ambient assisted living for people with motor impairments. In G. Kouroupetroglou (Ed.), *Disability informatics and web accessibility for motor limitations* (pp. 76–104). Hershey, PA: IGI Global. doi:10.4018/978-1-4666-4442-7.ch003

Adeyemo, O. (2013). The nationwide health information network: A biometric approach to prevent medical identity theft. In I. Management Association (Ed.), User-driven healthcare: Concepts, methodologies, tools, and applications (pp. 1636-1649). Hershey, PA: IGI Global. doi:10.4018/978-1-4666-2770-3.ch081

Åkerberg, A., Lindén, M., & Folke, M. (2013). Pedometer cell phone applications and future trends in measuring physical activity. In R. Martinho, R. Rijo, M. Cruz-Cunha, & J. Varajão (Eds.), *Information systems and technologies for enhancing health and social care* (pp. 324–339). Hershey, PA: IGI Global. doi:10.4018/978-1-4666-3667-5.ch021

Al Hamouche, V. (2014). Making quality control decisions in radiology department: A decision support system for radiographers' performance appraisal using PACS. In C. El Morr (Ed.), *Research perspectives on the role of informatics in health policy and management* (pp. 48–61). Hershey, PA: IGI Global. doi:10.4018/978-1-4666-4321-5.ch004

Al-Khudairy, S. (2014). Caring for our aging population: Using CPOE and telehomecare systems as a response to health policy concerns. In C. El Morr (Ed.), *Research perspectives on the role of informatics in health policy and management* (pp. 153–166). Hershey, PA: IGI Global. doi:10.4018/978-1-4666-4321-5.ch010

Albuquerque, C. (2013). The study of social needs as a strategic tool for the innovation of the social care sector: The contribution of new technologies. In M. Cruz-Cunha, I. Miranda, & P. Gonçalves (Eds.), *Handbook of research on ICTs for human-centered healthcare and social care services* (pp. 347–365). Hershey, PA: IGI Global. doi:10.4018/978-1-4666-3986-7.ch018

Alexandrou, D. A., & Pardalis, K. V. (2013). SEMantic PATHways: Modeling, executing, and monitoring intra-organizational healthcare business processes towards personalized treatment. In A. Moumtzoglou & A. Kastania (Eds.), *E-health technologies and improving patient safety: Exploring organizational factors* (pp. 98–123). Hershey, PA: IGI Global. doi:10.4018/978-1-4666-2657-7.ch007

Algarín, A. D., Demurjian, S. A., Ziminski, T. B., Sánchez, Y. K., & Kuykendall, R. (2014). Securing XML with role-based access control: Case study in health care. In A. Ruiz-Martinez, R. Marin-Lopez, & F. Pereniguez-Garcia (Eds.), *Architectures and protocols for secure information technology infrastructures* (pp. 334–365). Hershey, PA: IGI Global. doi:10.4018/978-1-4666-4514-1.ch013

Alhaqbani, B., & Fidge, C. (2013). A medical data trustworthiness assessment model. In I. Management Association (Ed.), *User-driven healthcare: Concepts, methodologies, tools, and applications* (pp. 1425-1445). Hershey, PA: IGI Global. doi:10.4018/978-1-4666-2770-3.ch071

Almeida, L., Menezes, P., & Dias, J. (2013). Augmented reality framework for the socialization between elderly people. In M. Cruz-Cunha, I. Miranda, & P. Gonçalves (Eds.), *Handbook of research on ICTs for human-centered healthcare and social care services* (pp. 430–448). Hershey, PA: IGI Global. doi:10.4018/978-1-4666-3986-7.ch023

Amer, M. B., Amawi, M., & El-Khatib, H. (2013). A novel neural fuzzy approach for diagnosis of potassium disturbances. In J. Tan (Ed.), *Healthcare information technology innovation and sustainability: Frontiers and adoption* (pp. 208–218). Hershey, PA: IGI Global. doi:10.4018/978-1-4666-2797-0.ch013

Andersen, S. T., & Jansen, A. (2013). Innovation in ICT-based health care provision. In J. Tan (Ed.), *Healthcare information technology innovation and sustainability: Frontiers and adoption* (pp. 58–72). Hershey, PA: IGI Global. doi:10.4018/978-1-4666-2797-0.ch004

Angjellari-Dajci, F., Lawless, W. F., Stachura, M. E., Wood, E. A., & DiBattisto, C. (2013). Economic evaluations for service delivery in autism spectrum disorders: benefit-cost analysis for emerging telehealth systems. In M. Cruz-Cunha, I. Miranda, & P. Gonçalves (Eds.), *Handbook of research on ICTs and management systems for improving efficiency in healthcare and social care* (pp. 16–42). Hershey, PA: IGI Global. doi:10.4018/978-1-4666-3990-4.ch002

Archibald, D., MacDonald, C. J., Hogue, R., & Mercer, J. (2013). Accessing knowledge from the bedside: Introducing the tablet computer to clinical teaching. In C. Rückemann (Ed.), *Integrated information and computing systems for natural, spatial, and social sciences* (pp. 96–109). Hershey, PA: IGI Global. doi:10.4018/978-1-4666-2190-9.ch005

Archondakis, S. (2013). Static telecytological applications for proficiency testing. In V. Gulla, A. Mori, F. Gabbrielli, & P. Lanzafame (Eds.), *Telehealth networks for hospital services: New methodologies* (pp. 228–239). Hershey, PA: IGI Global. doi:10.4018/978-1-4666-2979-0.ch015

Arling, P. A., Doebbeling, B. N., & Fox, R. L. (2013). Improving the implementation of evidence-based practice and information systems in healthcare: A social network approach. In J. Tan (Ed.), *Healthcare information technology innovation and sustainability: Frontiers and adoption* (pp. 247–270). Hershey, PA: IGI Global. doi:10.4018/978-1-4666-2797-0.ch016

Arriaga, P., Esteves, F., & Fernandes, S. (2013). Playing for better or for worse?: Health and social outcomes with electronic gaming. In M. Cruz-Cunha, I. Miranda, & P. Gonçalves (Eds.), *Handbook of research on ICTs for human-centered healthcare and social care services* (pp. 48–69). Hershey, PA: IGI Global. doi:10.4018/978-1-4666-3986-7.ch003

Arslan, P. (2014). Collaborative participation in personalized health through mobile diaries. In K. Rızvanoğlu & G. Çetin (Eds.), *Research and design innovations for mobile user experience* (pp. 150–181). Hershey, PA: IGI Global. doi:10.4018/978-1-4666-4446-5.ch009

Assis-Hassid, S., Reychav, I., Pliskin, J. S., & Heart, T. H. (2013). The effects of electronic medical record (EMR) use in primary care on the physician-patient relationship. In M. Cruz-Cunha, I. Miranda, & P. Gonçalves (Eds.), *Handbook of research on ICTs for human-centered healthcare and social care services* (pp. 130–150). Hershey, PA: IGI Global. doi:10.4018/978-1-4666-3986-7.ch007

Azar, A. T. (2013). Overview of biomedical engineering. In I. Management Association (Ed.), Bioinformatics: Concepts, methodologies, tools, and applications (pp. 1-28). Hershey, PA: IGI Global. doi:10.4018/978-1-4666-3604-0.ch001

Azar, A. T., & Eljamel, M. S. (2014). Medical robotics. In I. Management Association (Ed.), Robotics: Concepts, methodologies, tools, and applications (pp. 1116-1147). Hershey, PA: IGI Global. doi:10.4018/978-1-4666-4607-0.ch054

Baladrón, C., Aguiar, J. M., Calavia, L., Carro, B., & Sánchez-Esguevillas, A. (2014). Learning on the move in the web 2.0: New initiatives in m-learning. In *K-12 education: Concepts, methodologies, tools, and applications* (pp. 1693–1714). Hershey, PA: IGI Global. doi:10.4018/978-1-4666-4502-8.ch097

Bauer, K. A. (2013). Caught in the web: The internet and the demise of medical privacy. In I. Management Association (Ed.), User-driven healthcare: Concepts, methodologies, tools, and applications (pp. 1252-1272). Hershey, PA: IGI Global. doi:10.4018/978-1-4666-2770-3.ch063

Belsis, P., Skourlas, C., & Gritzalis, S. (2013). Secure electronic healthcare records management in wireless environments. In M. Khosrow-Pour (Ed.), *Interdisciplinary advances in information technology research* (pp. 202–219). Hershey, PA: IGI Global. doi:10.4018/978-1-4666-3625-5.ch015

Benito, R. V., Vega-Colado, C., Coco, M. B., Cuadrado, R., Torres-Zafra, J. C., Sánchez-Pena, J. M., ... López-Miguel, A. (2013). New electro-optic and display technology for visually disabled people. In M. Cruz-Cunha, I. Miranda, & P. Gonçalves (Eds.), *Handbook of research on ICTs for human-centered healthcare and social care services* (pp. 687–718). Hershey, PA: IGI Global. doi:10.4018/978-1-4666-3986-7.ch036

Bergenti, F., Poggi, A., & Tomaiuolo, M. (2013). Using multi-agent systems to support e-health services. In M. Cruz-Cunha, I. Miranda, & P. Gonçalves (Eds.), *Handbook of research on ICTs for human-centered healthcare and social care services* (pp. 549–567). Hershey, PA: IGI Global. doi:10.4018/978-1-4666-3986-7.ch029

Berler, A., & Apostolakis, I. (2014). Normalizing cross-border healthcare in Europe via new e-prescription paradigms. In C. El Morr (Ed.), *Research perspectives on the role of informatics in health policy and management* (pp. 168–208). Hershey, PA: IGI Global. doi:10.4018/978-1-4666-4321-5.ch011

Bernardi, R. (2013). Information technology and resistance to public sector reforms: A case study in Kenya. In I. Management Association (Ed.), User-driven healthcare: Concepts, methodologies, tools, and applications (pp. 14-33). Hershey, PA: IGI Global. doi:10.4018/978-1-4666-2770-3.ch002

Bernhard, S., Al Zoukra, K., & Schtte, C. (2013). From non-invasive hemodynamic measurements towards patient-specific cardiovascular diagnosis. In *Data mining: Concepts, methodologies, tools, and applications* (pp. 2069–2093). Hershey, PA: IGI Global. doi:10.4018/978-1-4666-2455-9.ch106

Best, C., O'Neill, B., & Gillespie, A. (2013). Assistive technology for cognition: Enabling activities of daily living. In M. Cruz-Cunha, I. Miranda, & P. Gonçalves (Eds.), *Handbook of research on ICTs for human-centered healthcare and social care services* (pp. 112–129). Hershey, PA: IGI Global. doi:10.4018/978-1-4666-3986-7.ch006

Bhattacharya, P., Asanga, A. P., & Biswas, R. (2013). Stomodeum to proctodeum: Email narratives on clinical problem solving in gastroenterology. In I. Management Association (Ed.), *User-driven healthcare: Concepts, methodologies, tools, and applications* (pp. 1073-1091). Hershey, PA: IGI Global. doi:10.4018/978-1-4666-2770-3.ch054

Boboc, C., & Ţiţan, E. (2014). Migration of medical doctors, health, medical education, and employment in eastern and central Europe. In A. Driouchi (Ed.), *Labor and health economics in the Mediterranean region: Migration and mobility of medical doctors* (pp. 158–191). Hershey, PA: IGI Global. doi:10.4018/978-1-4666-4723-7.ch007

Botella, C., Baños, R. M., Etchemendy, E., Castilla, D., García-Palacios, A., & Alcañiz, M. (2013). An e-health system for promoting wellbeing in the elderly: The butler system. In I. Management Association (Ed.), *User-driven healthcare: Concepts, methodologies, tools, and applications* (pp. 838-852). Hershey, PA: IGI Global. doi:10.4018/978-1-4666-2770-3.ch042

Bradai, N., Chaari, L., & Kamoun, L. (2013). A comprehensive overview of wireless body area networks (WBAN). In J. Rodrigues (Ed.), *Digital advances in medicine, e-health, and communication technologies* (pp. 1–32). Hershey, PA: IGI Global. doi:10.4018/978-1-4666-2794-9.ch001

Brown, K. E., Bayley, J., & Newby, K. (2013). Serious game for relationships and sex education: Application of an intervention mapping approach to development. In S. Arnab, I. Dunwell, & K. Debattista (Eds.), *Serious games for healthcare: Applications and implications* (pp. 135–166). Hershey, PA: IGI Global. doi:10.4018/978-1-4666-1903-6.ch007

Brown, M. (2013). Will comparative effectiveness research lead to healthcare rationing? In I. Management Association (Ed.), User-driven healthcare: Concepts, methodologies, tools, and applications (pp. 1487-1507). Hershey, PA: IGI Global. doi:10.4018/978-1-4666-2770-3.ch074

Burlamaqui, A. M., Azevedo, S. O., Silva, I. R., Silva, S. R., Souto da Silva, G. H., & Benjamim, X. C. … Felix de Castro, A. (2013). Low cost t-health and t-social with ginga: Experience with mime TV, ImFine, and iFunnyCube interactive TV programs. In M. Cruz-Cunha, I. Miranda, & P. Gonçalves (Eds.), Handbook of research on ICTs for human-centered healthcare and social care services (pp. 303-318). Hershey, PA: IGI Global. doi:10.4018/978-1-4666-3986-7.ch015

Burns, J., Blanchard, M., & Metcalf, A. (2013). Bridging the digital divide in Australia: The potential implications for the mental health of young people experiencing marginalisation. In *Digital literacy: Concepts, methodologies, tools, and applications* (pp. 772–793). Hershey, PA: IGI Global. doi:10.4018/978-1-4666-1852-7.ch040

Buyurgan, N., Rardin, R. L., Jayaraman, R., Varghese, V. M., & Burbano, A. (2013). A novel GS1 data standard adoption roadmap for healthcare providers. In J. Tan (Ed.), *Healthcare information technology innovation and sustainability: Frontiers and adoption* (pp. 41–57). Hershey, PA: IGI Global. doi:10.4018/978-1-4666-2797-0.ch003

Cabrita, M. D., & Cabrita, M. (2014). Applying social marketing to healthcare: Challenges and opportunities. In A. Kapoor & C. Kulshrestha (Eds.), *Dynamics of competitive advantage and consumer perception in social marketing* (pp. 78–97). Hershey, PA: IGI Global. doi:10.4018/978-1-4666-4430-4.ch004

Carroll, J. M., & Rosson, M. B. (2013). Community networks: Infrastructure and models for therapeutic support. In M. Cruz-Cunha, I. Miranda, & P. Gonçalves (Eds.), *Handbook of research on ICTs for human-centered healthcare and social care services* (pp. 187–207). Hershey, PA: IGI Global. doi:10.4018/978-1-4666-3986-7.ch010

Castiglioni, I., Gilardi, M. C., & Gallivanone, F. (2013). E-health decision support systems for the diagnosis of dementia diseases. In A. Moumtzoglou & A. Kastania (Eds.), *E-health technologies and improving patient safety: Exploring organizational factors* (pp. 84–97). Hershey, PA: IGI Global. doi:10.4018/978-1-4666-2657-7.ch006

Catley, C., Smith, K., McGregor, C., James, A., & Eklund, J. M. (2013). A framework for multidimensional real-time data analysis: A case study for the detection of apnoea of prematurity. In A. Gangopadhyay (Ed.), *Methods, models, and computation for medical informatics* (pp. 16–35). Hershey, PA: IGI Global. doi:10.4018/978-1-4666-2653-9.ch002

Chaari, L., & Kamoun, L. (2013). QoS concepts and architecture over wireless body area networks for healthcare applications. In J. Rodrigues (Ed.), *Digital advances in medicine, e-health, and communication technologies* (pp. 114–130). Hershey, PA: IGI Global. doi:10.4018/978-1-4666-2794-9.ch007

Chamberlin, B., Maloney, A., Gallagher, R. R., & Garza, M. L. (2013). Active video games: Potential for increased activity, suggestions for use, and guidelines for implementation. In S. Arnab, I. Dunwell, & K. Debattista (Eds.), *Serious games for healthcare: Applications and implications* (pp. 191–212). Hershey, PA: IGI Global. doi:10.4018/978-1-4666-1903-6.ch009

Charisi, A., Korvesis, P., & Megalooikonomou, V. (2013). Similarity searching of medical image data in distributed systems: Facilitating telemedicine applications. In A. Gangopadhyay (Ed.), *Methods, models, and computation for medical informatics* (pp. 58–77). Hershey, PA: IGI Global. doi:10.4018/978-1-4666-2653-9.ch004

Chattopadhyay, A., Malhotra, K., & Chatterjee, S. (2013). Ethical guidelines for the quality assessment of healthcare. In I. Management Association (Ed.), User-driven healthcare: Concepts, methodologies, tools, and applications (pp. 1332-1347). Hershey, PA: IGI Global. doi:10.4018/978-1-4666-2770-3.ch066

Chen, J. Y., Xu, H., Shi, P., Culbertson, A., & Meslin, E. M. (2013). Ethics and privacy considerations for systems biology applications in predictive and personalized medicine. In I. Management Association (Ed.), Bioinformatics: Concepts, methodologies, tools, and applications (pp. 1378-1404). Hershey, PA: IGI Global. doi:10.4018/978-1-4666-3604-0.ch071

Chen, Y. (2013). Construction of digital statistical atlases of the liver and their applications to computer-aided diagnosis. In J. Wu (Ed.), *Technological advancements in biomedicine for healthcare applications* (pp. 68–79). Hershey, PA: IGI Global. doi:10.4018/978-1-4666-2196-1.ch008

Cheng, B., Stanley, R. J., De, S., Antani, S., & Thoma, G. R. (2013). Automatic detection of arrow annotation overlays in biomedical images. In J. Tan (Ed.), *Healthcare information technology innovation and sustainability: Frontiers and adoption* (pp. 219–236). Hershey, PA: IGI Global. doi:10.4018/978-1-4666-2797-0.ch014

Cherian, E. J., & Ryan, T. W. (2014). Incongruent needs: Why differences in the iron-triangle of priorities make health information technology adoption and use difficult. In C. El Morr (Ed.), *Research perspectives on the role of informatics in health policy and management* (pp. 209–221). Hershey, PA: IGI Global. doi:10.4018/978-1-4666-4321-5.ch012

Chowdhry, N., Ashraf, A., Chowdhry, B., Baloch, A., Ansari, A., & De Meer, H. (2013). Grid for post operative care through wireless sensor networks. In I. Management Association (Ed.), User-driven healthcare: Concepts, methodologies, tools, and applications (pp. 514-531). Hershey, PA: IGI Global. doi:10.4018/978-1-4666-2770-3.ch026

Chun, S. A., Kwon, J. H., & Lee, H. (2013). Social credential-based role recommendation and patient privacy control in medical emergency. In A. Gangopadhyay (Ed.), *Methods, models, and computation for medical informatics* (pp. 215–237). Hershey, PA: IGI Global. doi:10.4018/978-1-4666-2653-9.ch013

Cohen, J. F., Bancilhon, J., & Sergay, S. (2013). An empirical study of patient willingness to use self-service technologies in the healthcare context. In M. Cruz-Cunha, I. Miranda, & P. Gonçalves (Eds.), *Handbook of research on ICTs and management systems for improving efficiency in healthcare and social care* (pp. 378–395). Hershey, PA: IGI Global. doi:10.4018/978-1-4666-3990-4.ch019

Constantinides, P. (2013). The development of the English national health information infrastructure. In I. Management Association (Ed.), *User-driven healthcare: Concepts, methodologies, tools, and applications* (pp. 968-991). Hershey, PA: IGI Global. doi:10.4018/978-1-4666-2770-3.ch049

Constantinides, P. (2013). The development of a regional health information infrastructure in Greece. In I. Management Association (Ed.), *User-driven healthcare: Concepts, methodologies, tools, and applications* (pp. 992-1017). Hershey, PA: IGI Global. doi:10.4018/978-1-4666-2770-3.ch050

Corrigan, D., Hederman, L., Khan, H., Taweel, A., Kostopoulou, O., & Delaney, B. (2013). An ontology-driven approach to clinical evidence modelling implementing clinical prediction rules. In A. Moumtzoglou & A. Kastania (Eds.), *E-health technologies and improving patient safety: Exploring organizational factors* (pp. 257–284). Hershey, PA: IGI Global. doi:10.4018/978-1-4666-2657-7.ch016

Corritore, C. L., Kracher, B., Wiedenbeck, S., & Marble, R. (2013). Foundations of trust for e-health. In I. Management Association (Ed.), *User-driven healthcare: Concepts, methodologies, tools, and applications* (pp. 1167-1193). Hershey, PA: IGI Global. doi:10.4018/978-1-4666-2770-3.ch059

Costa, Â., Andrade, F., & Novais, P. (2013). Privacy and data protection towards elderly healthcare. In M. Cruz-Cunha, I. Miranda, & P. Gonçalves (Eds.), *Handbook of research on ICTs for human-centered healthcare and social care services* (pp. 330–346). Hershey, PA: IGI Global. doi:10.4018/978-1-4666-3986-7.ch017

Coughlan, J., & Brinkman, W. (2013). Design considerations for delivering e-learning to surgical trainees. In J. Rodrigues (Ed.), *Digital advances in medicine, e-health, and communication technologies* (pp. 341–350). Hershey, PA: IGI Global. doi:10.4018/978-1-4666-2794-9.ch020

D'Abundo, M. L. (2013). Electronic health record implementation in the United States healthcare industry: Making the process of change manageable. In V. Wang (Ed.), *Handbook of research on technologies for improving the 21st century workforce: Tools for lifelong learning* (pp. 272–286). Hershey, PA: IGI Global. doi:10.4018/978-1-4666-2181-7.ch018

D'Abundo, M. L. (2013). Electronic health record implementation in the United States healthcare industry: Making the process of change manageable. In I. Management Association (Ed.), *User-driven healthcare: Concepts, methodologies, tools, and applications* (pp. 382-395). Hershey, PA: IGI Global. doi:10.4018/978-1-4666-2770-3.ch019

D'Andrea, A., Ferri, F., & Grifoni, P. (2013). RFID technologies in the health sector. In A. Moumtzoglou & A. Kastania (Eds.), *E-health technologies and improving patient safety: Exploring organizational factors* (pp. 140–147). Hershey, PA: IGI Global. doi:10.4018/978-1-4666-2657-7.ch009

D'Astolfo, C. (2014). Investing in a "rehabilitation model" to improve the decision-making process in long-term care. In C. El Morr (Ed.), *Research perspectives on the role of informatics in health policy and management* (pp. 37–47). Hershey, PA: IGI Global. doi:10.4018/978-1-4666-4321-5.ch003

Daniel, V. M. (2013). Genomics and genetic engineering: Playing God? In I. Management Association (Ed.), *Bioinformatics: Concepts, methodologies, tools, and applications* (pp. 249-267). Hershey, PA: IGI Global. doi:10.4018/978-1-4666-3604-0.ch013

Dasgupta, S. S. (2013). Cyber capability framework: A tool to evaluate ICT for development projects. In M. Cruz-Cunha, I. Miranda, & P. Gonçalves (Eds.), *Handbook of research on ICTs for human-centered healthcare and social care services* (pp. 399–406). Hershey, PA: IGI Global. doi:10.4018/978-1-4666-3986-7.ch021

Davis, S. A. (2013). Global telemedicine and ehealth: Advances for future healthcare – Using a systems approach to integrate healthcare functions. In V. Gulla, A. Mori, F. Gabbrielli, & P. Lanzafame (Eds.), *Telehealth networks for hospital services: New methodologies* (pp. 15–32). Hershey, PA: IGI Global. doi:10.4018/978-1-4666-2979-0.ch002

Deng, M., Petkovic, M., Nalin, M., & Baroni, I. (2013). Home healthcare in cloud computing. In M. Cruz-Cunha, I. Miranda, & P. Gonçalves (Eds.), *Handbook of research on ICTs and management systems for improving efficiency in healthcare and social care* (pp. 614–634). Hershey, PA: IGI Global. doi:10.4018/978-1-4666-3990-4.ch032

DeVany, M., Knobloch-Ludwig, K., Penticoff, M., Assimacopoulos, A., & Speedie, S. (2013). Telehealth implementation: The voice of experience. In S. Sarnikar, D. Bennett, & M. Gaynor (Eds.), *Cases on healthcare information technology for patient care management* (pp. 126–139). Hershey, PA: IGI Global. doi:10.4018/978-1-4666-2671-3.ch008

Ding, W., Qiu, P., Liu, Y., & Feng, W. (2013). Current omics technologies in biomarker discovery. In I. Management Association (Ed.), *Bioinformatics: Concepts, methodologies, tools, and applications* (pp. 465-497). Hershey, PA: IGI Global. doi:10.4018/978-1-4666-3604-0.ch027

Dingli, A., Abela, C., & D'Ambrogio, I. (2013). PINATA: Taking e-health a step forward. In A. Moumtzoglou & A. Kastania (Eds.), *E-health technologies and improving patient safety: Exploring organizational factors* (pp. 173–195). Hershey, PA: IGI Global. doi:10.4018/978-1-4666-2657-7.ch012

Dogra, D. P., Nandam, K., Majumdar, A. K., Sural, S., Mukhopadhyay, J., Majumdar, B., ... Mukherjee, S. (2013). A tool for automatic hammersmith infant neurological examination. In J. Rodrigues (Ed.), *Digital advances in medicine, e-health, and communication technologies* (pp. 301–311). Hershey, PA: IGI Global. doi:10.4018/978-1-4666-2794-9.ch017

Doyle, J., Bertolotto, M., & Wilson, D. (2013). Towards multimodal mobile GIS for the elderly. In *Digital literacy: Concepts, methodologies, tools, and applications* (pp. 590–609). Hershey, PA: IGI Global. doi:10.4018/978-1-4666-1852-7.ch031

Dragoni, A. F. (2013). Health services through digital terrestrial television. In V. Gulla, A. Mori, F. Gabbrielli, & P. Lanzafame (Eds.), *Telehealth networks for hospital services: New methodologies* (pp. 207–227). Hershey, PA: IGI Global. doi:10.4018/978-1-4666-2979-0.ch014

Dragoni, A. F. (2013). Virtual carer: A first prototype. In V. Gulla, A. Mori, F. Gabbrielli, & P. Lanzafame (Eds.), *Telehealth networks for hospital services: New methodologies* (pp. 290–299). Hershey, PA: IGI Global. doi:10.4018/978-1-4666-2979-0.ch019

Driouchi, A. (2014). Introduction to labor and health economics: Mobility of medical doctors in the Mediterranean region. In A. Driouchi (Ed.), *Labor and health economics in the Mediterranean region: Migration and mobility of medical doctors* (pp. 1–22). Hershey, PA: IGI Global. doi:10.4018/978-1-4666-4723-7.ch001

Driouchi, A. (2014). Medical knowledge, north-south cooperation, and mobility of medical doctors. In A. Driouchi (Ed.), *Labor and health economics in the Mediterranean region: Migration and mobility of medical doctors* (pp. 376–395). Hershey, PA: IGI Global. doi:10.4018/978-1-4666-4723-7.ch015

Driouchi, A. (2014). Skilled human resources in the health sectors and impacts of new health technologies on health workforce in developing economies. In A. Driouchi (Ed.), *Labor and health economics in the Mediterranean region: Migration and mobility of medical doctors* (pp. 23–50). Hershey, PA: IGI Global. doi:10.4018/978-1-4666-4723-7.ch002

Duan, X., Wang, X., & Huang, Q. (2013). Medical manipulators for surgical applications. In J. Wu (Ed.), *Technological advancements in biomedicine for healthcare applications* (pp. 111–122). Hershey, PA: IGI Global. doi:10.4018/978-1-4666-2196-1.ch012

Dugdale, A. (2013). Australian patient organizations: Using digital technologies to engage health citizen communities in health policy. In I. Management Association (Ed.), User-driven healthcare: Concepts, methodologies, tools, and applications (pp. 853-869). Hershey, PA: IGI Global. doi:10.4018/978-1-4666-2770-3.ch043

Dunwell, I., & Jarvis, S. (2013). A serious game for on-the-ward infection control awareness training: Ward off infection. In S. Arnab, I. Dunwell, & K. Debattista (Eds.), *Serious games for healthcare: Applications and implications* (pp. 233–246). Hershey, PA: IGI Global. doi:10.4018/978-1-4666-1903-6.ch011

Durant, K. T., McCray, A. T., & Safran, C. (2013). Identifying temporal changes and topics that promote growth within online communities: A prospective study of six online cancer forums. In A. Gangopadhyay (Ed.), *Methods, models, and computation for medical informatics* (pp. 78–97). Hershey, PA: IGI Global. doi:10.4018/978-1-4666-2653-9.ch005

El-Farargy, N. (2013). Refresher training in clinical psychology supervision: A blended learning approach. In A. Benson, J. Moore, & S. Williams van Rooij (Eds.), *Cases on educational technology planning, design, and implementation: A project management perspective* (pp. 295–317). Hershey, PA: IGI Global. doi:10.4018/978-1-4666-4237-9.ch016

Enquist, H. (2013). From idea to use: lessons learned from a participatory ICT healthcare case study. In I. Management Association (Ed.), User-driven healthcare: Concepts, methodologies, tools, and applications (pp. 1037-1053). Hershey, PA: IGI Global. doi:10.4018/978-1-4666-2770-3.ch052

Ervin, K. (2014). Legal and ethical considerations in the implementation of electronic health records. In J. Krueger (Ed.), *Cases on electronic records and resource management implementation in diverse environments* (pp. 193–210). Hershey, PA: IGI Global. doi:10.4018/978-1-4666-4466-3.ch012

Escayola, J., Trigo, J., Martínez, I., Martínez-Espronceda, M., Aragüés, A., Sancho, D., . . . García, J. (2013). Overview of the ISO/IEEE11073 family of standards and their applications to health monitoring. In I. Management Association (Ed.), User-driven healthcare: Concepts, methodologies, tools, and applications (pp. 357-381). Hershey, PA: IGI Global. doi:10.4018/978-1-4666-2770-3.ch018

Facelli, J. C., Hurdle, J. F., & Mitchell, J. A. (2013). Medical informatics and bioinformatics. In I. Management Association (Ed.), Bioinformatics: Concepts, methodologies, tools, and applications (pp. 195-221). Hershey, PA: IGI Global. doi:10.4018/978-1-4666-3604-0.ch010

Fakhar, A. (2014). Beyond brain drain: A case study of the benefits of cooperation on medical immigration. In A. Driouchi (Ed.), *Labor and health economics in the Mediterranean region: Migration and mobility of medical doctors* (pp. 294–313). Hershey, PA: IGI Global. doi:10.4018/978-1-4666-4723-7.ch012

Falan, S. L., Han, B., Zoeller, L. H., Tarn, J. M., & Roach, D. M. (2013). Sustaining healthcare through waste elimination: A taxonomic analysis with case illustrations. In J. Tan (Ed.), *Healthcare information technology innovation and sustainability: Frontiers and adoption* (pp. 18–39). Hershey, PA: IGI Global. doi:10.4018/978-1-4666-2797-0.ch002

Farinha, C., & Mira da Silva, M. (2013). Identifying requirements for healthcare information systems with focus groups. In M. Cruz-Cunha, I. Miranda, & P. Gonçalves (Eds.), *Handbook of research on ICTs for human-centered healthcare and social care services* (pp. 491–510). Hershey, PA: IGI Global. doi:10.4018/978-1-4666-3986-7.ch026

Fernando, J. (2013). The protocols of privileged information handling in an e-health context: Australia. In I. Management Association (Ed.), User-driven healthcare: Concepts, methodologies, tools, and applications (pp. 737-759). Hershey, PA: IGI Global. doi:10.4018/978-1-4666-2770-3.ch036

Ferreira, L., Teixeira, A., & Cunha, J. P. (2013). Medical information extraction in European Portuguese. In M. Cruz-Cunha, I. Miranda, & P. Gonçalves (Eds.), *Handbook of research on ICTs for human-centered healthcare and social care services* (pp. 607–626). Hershey, PA: IGI Global. doi:10.4018/978-1-4666-3986-7.ch032

Fitzpatrick, J. (2013). An exploration of the experiences of migrant women: Implications for policy development of effective user driven health care delivery systems. In I. Management Association (Ed.), User-driven healthcare: Concepts, methodologies, tools, and applications (pp. 954-967). Hershey, PA: IGI Global. doi:10.4018/978-1-4666-2770-3.ch048

Fitzpatrick, J., & Ako, W. (2013). Developing community ontologies in user driven healthcare. In I. Management Association (Ed.), User-driven healthcare: Concepts, methodologies, tools, and applications (pp. 655-672). Hershey, PA: IGI Global. doi:10.4018/978-1-4666-2770-3.ch032

Flores, A. E., Win, K. T., & Susilo, W. (2013). Secure exchange of electronic health records. In I. Management Association (Ed.), IT policy and ethics: Concepts, methodologies, tools, and applications (pp. 1059-1079). Hershey, PA: IGI Global. doi:10.4018/978-1-4666-2919-6.ch048

Flores, A. E., Win, K. T., & Susilo, W. (2013). Secure exchange of electronic health records. In I. Management Association (Ed.), User-driven healthcare: Concepts, methodologies, tools, and applications (pp. 1403-1424). Hershey, PA: IGI Global. doi:10.4018/978-1-4666-2770-3.ch070

Forrestal, E. J., Cellucci, L. W., Zeng, X., Kennedy, M. H., & Smith, D. (2013). Health information technology collaboration in community health centers: The community partners HealthNet, Inc. In S. Sarnikar, D. Bennett, & M. Gaynor (Eds.), *Cases on healthcare information technology for patient care management* (pp. 171–196). Hershey, PA: IGI Global. doi:10.4018/978-1-4666-2671-3.ch011

Frederico, C. (2013). Nutrition games. In S. Arnab, I. Dunwell, & K. Debattista (Eds.), *Serious games for healthcare: Applications and implications* (pp. 167–190). Hershey, PA: IGI Global. doi:10.4018/978-1-4666-1903-6.ch008

Freitas, L., Pereira, R. T., Pereira, H. G., Martini, R., Mozzaquatro, B. A., Kasper, J., & Librelotto, G. (2013). Ontological representation and an architecture for homecare pervasive systems. In R. Martinho, R. Rijo, M. Cruz-Cunha, & J. Varajão (Eds.), *Information systems and technologies for enhancing health and social care* (pp. 215–234). Hershey, PA: IGI Global. doi:10.4018/978-1-4666-3667-5.ch015

Frigo, C. A., & Pavan, E. E. (2014). Prosthetic and orthotic devices. In *Assistive technologies: Concepts, methodologies, tools, and applications* (pp. 549–613). Hershey, PA: IGI Global. doi:10.4018/978-1-4666-4422-9.ch028

Fukami, T., & Wu, J. (2013). Image fusion method and the efficacy of multimodal cardiac images. In J. Wu (Ed.), *Technological advancements in biomedicine for healthcare applications* (pp. 47–54). Hershey, PA: IGI Global. doi:10.4018/978-1-4666-2196-1.ch006

Furdu, I., & Patrut, B. (2013). ICT applications and solutions in healthcare: Present and perspectives. In M. Cruz-Cunha, I. Miranda, & P. Gonçalves (Eds.), *Handbook of research on ICTs and management systems for improving efficiency in healthcare and social care* (pp. 559–576). Hershey, PA: IGI Global. doi:10.4018/978-1-4666-3990-4.ch029

Gabbrielli, F. (2013). Telemedicine R&D influencing incoming strategies and organization models. In V. Gulla, A. Mori, F. Gabbrielli, & P. Lanzafame (Eds.), *Telehealth networks for hospital services: New methodologies* (pp. 250–264). Hershey, PA: IGI Global. doi:10.4018/978-1-4666-2979-0.ch017

Gaivéo, J. M. (2013). Security of ICTs supporting healthcare activities. In M. Cruz-Cunha, I. Miranda, & P. Gonçalves (Eds.), *Handbook of research on ICTs for human-centered healthcare and social care services* (pp. 208–228). Hershey, PA: IGI Global. doi:10.4018/978-1-4666-3986-7.ch011

Gallo, C. (2013). A multichannel framework for multimedia content deployment in e-health environments. In M. Cruz-Cunha, I. Miranda, & P. Gonçalves (Eds.), *Handbook of research on ICTs and management systems for improving efficiency in healthcare and social care* (pp. 872–891). Hershey, PA: IGI Global. doi:10.4018/978-1-4666-3990-4.ch045

Gao, Y., Yang, W., Yang, J., Satoshi, T., & Wu, J. (2013). Neural mechanisms of audiovisual integration in integrated processing for verbal perception and spatial factors. In J. Wu (Ed.), *Biomedical engineering and cognitive neuroscience for healthcare: Interdisciplinary applications* (pp. 327–336). Hershey, PA: IGI Global. doi:10.4018/978-1-4666-2113-8.ch034

Garzo, A., Carmien, S. P., & Madina, X. (2013). Mapping input technology to ability. In I. Management Association (Ed.), User-driven healthcare: Concepts, methodologies, tools, and applications (pp. 480-501). Hershey, PA: IGI Global. doi:10.4018/978-1-4666-2770-3.ch024

Gatzidis, C. (2013). First-person shooter game engines and healthcare: An examination of the current state of the art and future potential. In S. Arnab, I. Dunwell, & K. Debattista (Eds.), *Serious Games for Healthcare: Applications and Implications* (pp. 76–89). Hershey, PA: IGI Global. doi:10.4018/978-1-4666-1903-6.ch004

Gaughan, M. (2013). The hybridized nature of America's health care system: Medicare as a case of both market and public failure. In M. Merviö (Ed.), *Healthcare management and economics: Perspectives on public and private administration* (pp. 154–164). Hershey, PA: IGI Global. doi:10.4018/978-1-4666-3982-9.ch012

Gavgani, V. Z. (2013). Information therapy (ix) service and patients' preference. In A. Gangopadhyay (Ed.), *Methods, models, and computation for medical informatics* (pp. 117–125). Hershey, PA: IGI Global. doi:10.4018/978-1-4666-2653-9.ch007

Gavgani, V. Z. (2013). Ubiquitous information therapy service through social networking libraries: An operational web 2.0 service model. In I. Management Association (Ed.), User-driven healthcare: Concepts, methodologies, tools, and applications (pp. 673-688). Hershey, PA: IGI Global. doi:10.4018/978-1-4666-2770-3.ch033

Germaine-McDaniel, N. S. (2013). The emerging hispanic use of online health information in the United States: Cultural convergence or dissociation? In I. Management Association (Ed.), User-driven healthcare: Concepts, methodologies, tools, and applications (pp. 1607-1621). Hershey, PA: IGI Global. doi:10.4018/978-1-4666-2770-3.ch079

Gholson, J., & Tennyson, H. (2013). One system of care, one electronic chart. In S. Sarnikar, D. Bennett, & M. Gaynor (Eds.), *Cases on healthcare information technology for patient care management* (pp. 55–69). Hershey, PA: IGI Global. doi:10.4018/978-1-4666-2671-3.ch003

Ghosh, B. (2013). Healthcare systems using clinical data: Addressing data interoperability challenges. In S. Sarnikar, D. Bennett, & M. Gaynor (Eds.), *Cases on healthcare information technology for patient care management* (pp. 208–223). Hershey, PA: IGI Global. doi:10.4018/978-1-4666-2671-3.ch013

Gibson, L., Sloan, D., & Moncur, W. (2013). E-health and digital inclusion. In I. Management Association (Ed.), User-driven healthcare: Concepts, methodologies, tools, and applications (pp. 197-210). Hershey, PA: IGI Global. doi:10.4018/978-1-4666-2770-3.ch011

Gillies, A. C., & Howard, J. (2013). Information as change agent or barrier in health care reform? In J. Tan (Ed.), *Healthcare information technology innovation and sustainability: Frontiers and adoption* (pp. 1–17). Hershey, PA: IGI Global. doi:10.4018/978-1-4666-2797-0.ch001

Glusker, A., & Hoelscher, E. (2014). Transitioning from print to online-only resources: The experience of a medium-sized healthcare organization library. In J. Krueger (Ed.), *Cases on electronic records and resource management implementation in diverse environments* (pp. 226–242). Hershey, PA: IGI Global. doi:10.4018/978-1-4666-4466-3.ch014

Gofuku, A., Fukumori, S., & Sato, K. (2013). A mirror visual feedback therapy system applying virtual reality technology. In J. Wu (Ed.), *Biomedical engineering and cognitive neuroscience for healthcare: Interdisciplinary applications* (pp. 73–80). Hershey, PA: IGI Global. doi:10.4018/978-1-4666-2113-8.ch008

Gomes, C., Sperandio, F., Peles, A., Borges, J., Brito, A. C., & Almada-Lobo, B. (2013). An operating theater planning decision support system. In R. Martinho, R. Rijo, M. Cruz-Cunha, & J. Varajão (Eds.), *Information systems and technologies for enhancing health and social care* (pp. 69–86). Hershey, PA: IGI Global. doi:10.4018/978-1-4666-3667-5.ch005

Grissom, T. E., DuKatz, A., Kordylewski, H. A., & Dutton, R. P. (2013). Bring out your data: The evolution of the national anesthesia clinical outcomes registry (NACOR). In A. Gangopadhyay (Ed.), *Methods, models, and computation for medical informatics* (pp. 126–145). Hershey, PA: IGI Global. doi:10.4018/978-1-4666-2653-9.ch008

Gudes, O., Kendall, E., Yigitcanlar, T., Han, J. H., & Pathak, V. (2013). Developing a competitive city through healthy decision-making. In I. Management Association (Ed.), User-driven healthcare: Concepts, methodologies, tools, and applications (pp. 808-822). Hershey, PA: IGI Global. doi:10.4018/978-1-4666-2770-3.ch040

Gugerty, B., & Maranda, M. J. (2013). The promises and challenges of health information technology. In I. Management Association (Ed.), User-driven healthcare: Concepts, methodologies, tools, and applications (pp. 57-76). Hershey, PA: IGI Global. doi:10.4018/978-1-4666-2770-3.ch004

Guimarães, C., Antunes, D. R., García, L. S., & Fernandes, S. (2013). Information challenges of the deaf in their health and social care needs. In M. Cruz-Cunha, I. Miranda, & P. Gonçalves (Eds.), *Handbook of research on ICTs for human-centered healthcare and social care services* (pp. 93–111). Hershey, PA: IGI Global. doi:10.4018/978-1-4666-3986-7.ch005

Guinalíu, M., Marta, J., & Subero, J. M. (2013). Social networks as a tool to improve the life quality of chronic patients and their relatives. In M. Cruz-Cunha, I. Miranda, & P. Gonçalves (Eds.), *Handbook of research on ICTs for human-centered healthcare and social care services* (pp. 172–186). Hershey, PA: IGI Global. doi:10.4018/978-1-4666-3986-7.ch009

Gullà, V. (2013). Leading the technological innovation in healthcare systems: The telematic medicine approach. In V. Gulla, A. Mori, F. Gabbrielli, & P. Lanzafame (Eds.), *Telehealth networks for hospital services: New methodologies* (pp. 134–153). Hershey, PA: IGI Global. doi:10.4018/978-1-4666-2979-0.ch009

Gullà, V., & Cancellotti, C. (2013). Telemedicine in emergency: A first aid hospital network experience. In V. Gulla, A. Mori, F. Gabbrielli, & P. Lanzafame (Eds.), *Telehealth networks for hospital services: New methodologies* (pp. 240–248). Hershey, PA: IGI Global. doi:10.4018/978-1-4666-2979-0.ch016

Guo, M., Yu, Y., Yang, J., & Wu, J. (2013). The crossmodal between the visual and tactile for motion perception. In J. Wu (Ed.), *Biomedical engineering and cognitive neuroscience for healthcare: Interdisciplinary applications* (pp. 99–108). Hershey, PA: IGI Global. doi:10.4018/978-1-4666-2113-8.ch011

Habib, M. K. (2014). Web-based multi-user distributed and collaborative environment supporting emergency and relief activities. In I. Management Association (Ed.), Crisis management: Concepts, methodologies, tools and applications (pp. 425-445). Hershey, PA: IGI Global. doi:10.4018/978-1-4666-4707-7.ch019

Hafeez-Baig, A., & Gururajan, R. (2013). Phenomena of adoption of wireless handheld devices: A case of healthcare setting. In H. Muga & K. Thomas (Eds.), *Cases on the diffusion and adoption of sustainable development practices* (pp. 20–43). Hershey, PA: IGI Global. doi:10.4018/978-1-4666-2842-7.ch002

Haida, M. (2013). Implications of NIRS brain signals. In J. Wu (Ed.), *Biomedical engineering and cognitive neuroscience for healthcare: Interdisciplinary applications* (pp. 120–128). Hershey, PA: IGI Global. doi:10.4018/978-1-4666-2113-8.ch013

Han, D., & Braun, K. L. (2013). Promoting active ageing through technology training in Korea. In *Digital literacy: Concepts, methodologies, tools, and applications* (pp. 572–589). Hershey, PA: IGI Global. doi:10.4018/978-1-4666-1852-7.ch030

Haniff, D. (2013). Usability engineering and e-health. In I. Management Association (Ed.), User-driven healthcare: Concepts, methodologies, tools, and applications (pp. 1446-1468). Hershey, PA: IGI Global. doi:10.4018/978-1-4666-2770-3.ch072

Hareva, D. H., Okada, H., & Oka, H. (2013). Ecological momentary assessment using a mobile phone. In J. Wu (Ed.), *Technological advancements in biomedicine for healthcare applications* (pp. 398–407). Hershey, PA: IGI Global. doi:10.4018/978-1-4666-2196-1.ch039

Harnett, B. (2013). Patient centered medicine and technology adaptation. In I. Management Association (Ed.), User-driven healthcare: Concepts, methodologies, tools, and applications (pp. 77-98). Hershey, PA: IGI Global. doi:10.4018/978-1-4666-2770-3.ch005

Hatton, J. D., Schmidt, T. M., & Jelen, J. (2013). Adoption of electronic health care records: Physician heuristics and hesitancy. In R. Martinho, R. Rijo, M. Cruz-Cunha, & J. Varajão (Eds.), *Information systems and technologies for enhancing health and social care* (pp. 148–165). Hershey, PA: IGI Global. doi:10.4018/978-1-4666-3667-5.ch010

Heinrichs, L., Fellander-Tsai, L., & Davies, D. (2013). Clinical virtual worlds: The wider implications for professional development in healthcare. In K. Bredl & W. Bösche (Eds.), *Serious games and virtual worlds in education, professional development, and healthcare* (pp. 221–240). Hershey, PA: IGI Global. doi:10.4018/978-1-4666-3673-6.ch014

Heinrichs, W. L., Davies, D., & Davies, J. (2013). Virtual worlds in healthcare: Applications and implications. In S. Arnab, I. Dunwell, & K. Debattista (Eds.), *Serious games for healthcare: Applications and implications* (pp. 1–22). Hershey, PA: IGI Global. doi:10.4018/978-1-4666-1903-6.ch001

Hirata, M., Yanagisawa, T., Matsushita, K., Sugata, H., Kamitani, Y., & Suzuki, T. ... Yoshimine, T. (2013). Brain–machine interface using brain surface electrodes: Real-time robotic control and a fully implantable wireless system. In J. Wu (Ed.), Technological advancements in biomedicine for healthcare applications (pp. 362-374). Hershey, PA: IGI Global. doi:10.4018/978-1-4666-2196-1.ch036

Hocine, N., & Gouaïch, A. (2013). Difficulty and scenario adaptation: An approach to customize therapeutic games. In S. Arnab, I. Dunwell, & K. Debattista (Eds.), *Serious games for healthcare: Applications and implications* (pp. 107–134). Hershey, PA: IGI Global. doi:10.4018/978-1-4666-1903-6.ch006

Hoonakker, P., Cartmill, R. S., Carayon, P., & Walker, J. M. (2013). Development and psychometric qualities of the SEIPS survey to evaluate CPOE/EHR implementation in ICUs. In J. Tan (Ed.), *Healthcare information technology innovation and sustainability: Frontiers and adoption* (pp. 161–179). Hershey, PA: IGI Global. doi:10.4018/978-1-4666-2797-0.ch010

Hoshi, K. (2013). Reframing dichotomies: Human experiential design of healthcare technologies. In I. Management Association (Ed.), User-driven healthcare: Concepts, methodologies, tools, and applications (pp. 1303-1331). Hershey, PA: IGI Global. doi:10.4018/978-1-4666-2770-3.ch065

Høstgaard, A. M. (2013). End-user participation in health IT development: The EUPHIT method. In I. Management Association (Ed.), User-driven healthcare: Concepts, methodologies, tools, and applications (pp. 608-629). Hershey, PA: IGI Global. doi:10.4018/978-1-4666-2770-3.ch030

Igrejas, G., Amaral, J. S., & Rodrigues, P. J. (2013). Fall detection systems to be used by elderly people. In M. Cruz-Cunha, I. Miranda, & P. Gonçalves (Eds.), *Handbook of research on ICTs for human-centered healthcare and social care services* (pp. 449–473). Hershey, PA: IGI Global. doi:10.4018/978-1-4666-3986-7.ch024

Inomata, C., & Nitta, S. (2013). Nursing in integrative medicine and nurses' engagement in caring-healing: A discussion based on the practice and study of music therapy and nursing care for patients with neurodegenerative disorders. In J. Wu (Ed.), *Technological advancements in biomedicine for healthcare applications* (pp. 235–239). Hershey, PA: IGI Global. doi:10.4018/978-1-4666-2196-1.ch025

Ishaq, G. M., Hussain, P. T., Iqbal, M. J., & Mushtaq, M. B. (2013). Risk-benefit analysis of combination vs. unopposed HRT in post-menopausal women. In I. Management Association (Ed.), Bioinformatics: Concepts, methodologies, tools, and applications (pp. 1424-1440). Hershey, PA: IGI Global. doi:10.4018/978-1-4666-3604-0.ch073

Iwaki, S. (2013). Multimodal neuroimaging to visualize human visual processing. In J. Wu (Ed.), *Biomedical engineering and cognitive neuroscience for healthcare: Interdisciplinary applications* (pp. 274–282). Hershey, PA: IGI Global. doi:10.4018/978-1-4666-2113-8.ch028

Ji, Z., Sugi, T., Goto, S., Wang, X., & Nakamura, M. (2013). Multi-channel template extraction for automatic EEG spike detection. In J. Wu (Ed.), *Biomedical engineering and cognitive neuroscience for healthcare: Interdisciplinary applications* (pp. 255–265). Hershey, PA: IGI Global. doi:10.4018/978-1-4666-2113-8.ch026

Jiang, Y., Wang, S., Tan, R., Ishida, K., Ando, T., & Fujie, M. G. (2013). Motor cortex activation during mental imagery of walking: An fNIRS study. In J. Wu (Ed.), *Biomedical engineering and cognitive neuroscience for healthcare: Interdisciplinary applications* (pp. 29–37). Hershey, PA: IGI Global. doi:10.4018/978-1-4666-2113-8.ch004

Johnson, K., & Tashiro, J. (2013). Interprofessional care and health care complexity: Factors shaping human resources effectiveness in health information management. In I. Management Association (Ed.), User-Driven Healthcare: Concepts, Methodologies, Tools, and Applications (pp. 1273-1302). Hershey, PA: IGI Global. doi:10.4018/978-1-4666-2770-3.ch064

Jose, J. (2013). Pharmacovigilance: Basic concepts and applications of pharmacoinformatics. In I. Management Association (Ed.), Bioinformatics: Concepts, methodologies, tools, and applications (pp. 1453-1473). Hershey, PA: IGI Global. doi:10.4018/978-1-4666-3604-0.ch075

Kalina, J., & Zvárová, J. (2013). Decision support systems in the process of improving patient safety. In A. Moumtzoglou & A. Kastania (Eds.), *E-health technologies and improving patient safety: Exploring organizational factors* (pp. 71–83). Hershey, PA: IGI Global. doi:10.4018/978-1-4666-2657-7.ch005

Kalina, J., & Zvárová, J. (2013). Decision support systems in the process of improving patient safety. In I. Management Association (Ed.), Bioinformatics: Concepts, methodologies, tools, and applications (pp. 1113-1125). Hershey, PA: IGI Global. doi:10.4018/978-1-4666-3604-0.ch057

Kamath, J. R., & Donahoe-Anshus, A. L. (2013). Electronic health record: Adoption, considerations and future direction. In I. Management Association (Ed.), User-driven healthcare: Concepts, methodologies, tools, and applications (pp. 34-56). Hershey, PA: IGI Global. doi:10.4018/978-1-4666-2770-3.ch003

Karamagkioli, K. Z., & Karamagioli, E. (2013). European e-health framework: Towards more "patient-friendly" healthcare services? In I. Management Association (Ed.), User-driven healthcare: Concepts, methodologies, tools, and applications (pp. 760-775). Hershey, PA: IGI Global. doi:10.4018/978-1-4666-2770-3.ch037

Kardaras, D. K., & Karakostas, B. (2013). Case studies in customization of e-health services. In I. Management Association (Ed.), User-driven healthcare: Concepts, methodologies, tools, and applications (pp. 1018-1036). Hershey, PA: IGI Global. doi:10.4018/978-1-4666-2770-3.ch051

Kastania, A. N. (2013). Evaluation considerations for e-health systems. In I. Management Association (Ed.), User-driven healthcare: Concepts, methodologies, tools, and applications (pp. 1126-1140). Hershey, PA: IGI Global. doi:10.4018/978-1-4666-2770-3.ch057

Kato, P. M. (2013). The role of the researcher in making serious games for health. In S. Arnab, I. Dunwell, & K. Debattista (Eds.), *Serious games for healthcare: Applications and implications* (pp. 213–231). Hershey, PA: IGI Global. doi:10.4018/978-1-4666-1903-6.ch010

Katsura, S. (2013). Preservation and reproduction of human motion based on a motion-copying system. In J. Wu (Ed.), *Technological advancements in biomedicine for healthcare applications* (pp. 375–384). Hershey, PA: IGI Global. doi:10.4018/978-1-4666-2196-1.ch037

Kikuchi, T. (2013). Human-friendly mechatronics systems with functional fluids and elastomers. In J. Wu (Ed.), *Technological advancements in biomedicine for healthcare applications* (pp. 94–101). Hershey, PA: IGI Global. doi:10.4018/978-1-4666-2196-1.ch010

Kimura, T., Miura, T., Shinohara, K., & Doi, S. (2013). Visual attention in 3-D space while moving forward. In J. Wu (Ed.), *Biomedical engineering and cognitive neuroscience for healthcare: Interdisciplinary applications* (pp. 81–88). Hershey, PA: IGI Global. doi:10.4018/978-1-4666-2113-8.ch009

Kldiashvili, E. (2013). Implementation of telecytology in Georgia. In V. Gulla, A. Mori, F. Gabbrielli, & P. Lanzafame (Eds.), *Telehealth networks for hospital services: New methodologies* (pp. 341–361). Hershey, PA: IGI Global. doi:10.4018/978-1-4666-2979-0.ch022

Kolovou, L. T., & Lymberopoulos, D. K. (2013). The concept of interoperability for AAL systems. In I. Management Association (Ed.), User-driven healthcare: Concepts, methodologies, tools, and applications (pp. 1364-1385). Hershey, PA: IGI Global. doi:10.4018/978-1-4666-2770-3.ch068

Koppar, A. R., & Sridhar, V. (2013). Malaria parasite detection: Automated method using microscope color image. In J. Rodrigues (Ed.), *Digital advances in medicine, e-health, and communication technologies* (pp. 289–300). Hershey, PA: IGI Global. doi:10.4018/978-1-4666-2794-9.ch016

Kotsonis, E., & Eliakis, S. (2013). Information security standards for health information systems: The implementer's approach. In I. Management Association (Ed.), User-driven healthcare: Concepts, methodologies, tools, and applications (pp. 225-257). Hershey, PA: IGI Global. doi:10.4018/978-1-4666-2770-3.ch013

Krishnaswamy, K., & Oates, T. (2014). Pathway to independence: Past, present, and beyond via robotics. In G. Kouroupetroglou (Ed.), *Disability informatics and web accessibility for motor limitations* (pp. 153–201). Hershey, PA: IGI Global. doi:10.4018/978-1-4666-4442-7.ch005

Kuehler, M., Schimke, N., & Hale, J. (2013). Privacy considerations for electronic health records. In I. Management Association (Ed.), User-driven healthcare: Concepts, methodologies, tools, and applications (pp. 1387-1402). Hershey, PA: IGI Global. doi:10.4018/978-1-4666-2770-3.ch069

Kurita, Y., Ikeda, A., Nagata, K., Okajima, M., & Ogasawara, T. (2013). Biomedical robotics for healthcare. In J. Wu (Ed.), *Technological advancements in biomedicine for healthcare applications* (pp. 160–169). Hershey, PA: IGI Global. doi:10.4018/978-1-4666-2196-1.ch017

Lakkaraju, S., & Lakkaraju, S. (2013). Mobile device application in healthcare. In S. Sarnikar, D. Bennett, & M. Gaynor (Eds.), *Cases on healthcare information technology for patient care management* (pp. 276–307). Hershey, PA: IGI Global. doi:10.4018/978-1-4666-2671-3.ch016

Laskowski, M. (2013). A prototype agent based model and machine learning hybrid system for healthcare decision support. In J. Rodrigues (Ed.), *Digital advances in medicine, e-health, and communication technologies* (pp. 230–253). Hershey, PA: IGI Global. doi:10.4018/978-1-4666-2794-9.ch013

Lee, T. (2014). Mobile healthcare computing in the cloud. In J. Rodrigues, K. Lin, & J. Lloret (Eds.), *Mobile networks and cloud computing convergence for progressive services and applications* (pp. 275–294). Hershey, PA: IGI Global. doi:10.4018/978-1-4666-4781-7.ch015

Lelardeux, C., Alvarez, J., Montaut, T., Galaup, M., & Lagarrigue, P. (2013). Healthcare games and the metaphoric approach. In S. Arnab, I. Dunwell, & K. Debattista (Eds.), *Serious games for healthcare: Applications and implications* (pp. 23–49). Hershey, PA: IGI Global. doi:10.4018/978-1-4666-1903-6.ch002

Lhotska, L., Bursa, M., Huptych, M., Chudacek, V., & Havlik, J. (2013). Interoperability of medical devices and information systems. In M. Cruz-Cunha, I. Miranda, & P. Gonçalves (Eds.), *Handbook of research on ICTs for human-centered healthcare and social care services* (pp. 749–762). Hershey, PA: IGI Global. doi:10.4018/978-1-4666-3986-7.ch039

Li, X., Lin, Z., & Wu, J. (2013). Language processing in the human brain of literate and illiterate subjects. In J. Wu (Ed.), *Biomedical engineering and cognitive neuroscience for healthcare: Interdisciplinary applications* (pp. 201–209). Hershey, PA: IGI Global. doi:10.4018/978-1-4666-2113-8.ch021

Liao, H. (2013). Biomedical information processing and visualization for minimally invasive neurosurgery. In J. Wu (Ed.), *Technological advancements in biomedicine for healthcare applications* (pp. 36–46). Hershey, PA: IGI Global. doi:10.4018/978-1-4666-2196-1.ch005

Libreri, C., & Graffigna, G. (2014). How web 2.0 shapes patient knowledge sharing: The case of diabetes in Italy. In C. El Morr (Ed.), *Research perspectives on the role of informatics in health policy and management* (pp. 238–260). Hershey, PA: IGI Global. doi:10.4018/978-1-4666-4321-5.ch014

Lin, C., Huang, Y., Li, C., & Jalleh, G. (2013). Key health information systems outsourcing issues from six hospital cases. In I. Management Association (Ed.), *User-driven healthcare: Concepts, methodologies, tools, and applications* (pp. 824-837). Hershey, PA: IGI Global. doi:10.4018/978-1-4666-2770-3.ch041

Lin, L., Chen, Y., Wu, J., & Tennyson, R. D. (2013). What skill/knowledge is important to a nursing professional? In P. Ordóñez de Pablos (Ed.), *Business, technology, and knowledge management in Asia: Trends and innovations* (pp. 234–249). Hershey, PA: IGI Global. doi:10.4018/978-1-4666-2652-2.ch018

Liu, G. (2014). Using case costing data and case mix for funding and benchmarking in rehabilitation hospitals. In C. El Morr (Ed.), *Research perspectives on the role of informatics in health policy and management* (pp. 62–78). Hershey, PA: IGI Global. doi:10.4018/978-1-4666-4321-5.ch005

Lixun, Z., Dapeng, B., & Lei, Y. (2013). Design of and experimentation with a walking assistance robot. In J. Wu (Ed.), *Technological advancements in biomedicine for healthcare applications* (pp. 123–127). Hershey, PA: IGI Global. doi:10.4018/978-1-4666-2196-1.ch013

Lui, K. (2013). The health informatics professional. In I. Management Association (Ed.), User-driven healthcare: Concepts, methodologies, tools, and applications (pp. 120-141). Hershey, PA: IGI Global. doi:10.4018/978-1-4666-2770-3.ch007

Ma, X., Chen, G., & Xiao, J. (2013). Understanding weight change behaviors through online social networks. In A. Gangopadhyay (Ed.), *Methods, models, and computation for medical informatics* (pp. 189–214). Hershey, PA: IGI Global. doi:10.4018/978-1-4666-2653-9.ch012

Makikawa, M., Okada, S., Fujiwara, Y., & Esaki, M. (2013). Sleep monitoring system equipped with a flexible non-contact ECG, respiration, and body motion sensor. In J. Wu (Ed.), *Technological advancements in biomedicine for healthcare applications* (pp. 287–297). Hershey, PA: IGI Global. doi:10.4018/978-1-4666-2196-1.ch030

Malindretos, G. (2013). Distribution and logistics outsourcing in the pharmaceutical sector. In D. Folinas (Ed.), *Outsourcing management for supply chain operations and logistics service* (pp. 202–222). Hershey, PA: IGI Global. doi:10.4018/978-1-4666-2008-7.ch012

Manvi, S. S., & B., M. R. (2013). A survey on health care services using wireless sensor networks. In M. Cruz-Cunha, I. Miranda, & P. Gonçalves (Eds.), *Handbook of research on ICTs for human-centered healthcare and social care services* (pp. 587-606). Hershey, PA: IGI Global. doi:10.4018/978-1-4666-3986-7.ch031

Marshall, S., & Hogan, J. (2013). The use of medical simulation to improve patient safety. In A. Moumtzoglou & A. Kastania (Eds.), *E-health technologies and improving patient safety: Exploring organizational factors* (pp. 155–172). Hershey, PA: IGI Global. doi:10.4018/978-1-4666-2657-7.ch011

Martin, J., & McKay, E. (2013). Mental health, post-secondary education, and information communications technology. In J. Lannon & E. Halpin (Eds.), *Human rights and information communication technologies: Trends and consequences of use* (pp. 196–213). Hershey, PA: IGI Global. doi:10.4018/978-1-4666-1918-0.ch012

Martin, J., & McKay, E. (2014). Mental health, post-secondary education, and information communications technology. In *Assistive technologies: Concepts, methodologies, tools, and applications* (pp. 1209–1226). Hershey, PA: IGI Global. doi:10.4018/978-1-4666-4422-9.ch063

Martin, V. (2013). Developing a library collection in bioinformatics: Support for an evolving profession. In I. Management Association (Ed.), Bioinformatics: Concepts, methodologies, tools, and applications (pp. 130-150). Hershey, PA: IGI Global. doi:10.4018/978-1-4666-3604-0.ch007

Masayuki, K., Eiji, K., Tetsuo, T., & Nozomu, M. (2013). Evaluation of olfactory impairment in Parkinson's disease using near-infrared spectroscopy. In J. Wu (Ed.), *Biomedical engineering and cognitive neuroscience for healthcare: Interdisciplinary applications* (pp. 293–302). Hershey, PA: IGI Global. doi:10.4018/978-1-4666-2113-8.ch030

Mazzanti, I., Maolo, A., & Antonicelli, R. (2013). E-health and telemedicine in the elderly: State of the art. In V. Gulla, A. Mori, F. Gabbrielli, & P. Lanzafame (Eds.), *Telehealth Networks for Hospital Services: New Methodologies* (pp. 33–43). Hershey, PA: IGI Global. doi:10.4018/978-1-4666-2979-0.ch003

Mazzanti, I., Maolo, A., & Antonicelli, R. (2014). E-health and telemedicine in the elderly: State of the art. In *Assistive technologies: Concepts, methodologies, tools, and applications* (pp. 693–704). Hershey, PA: IGI Global. doi:10.4018/978-1-4666-4422-9.ch034

McCrossan, B. A., & Casey, F. A. (2013). The role of telemedicine in paediatric cardiology. In V. Gulla, A. Mori, F. Gabbrielli, & P. Lanzafame (Eds.), *Telehealth networks for hospital services: New methodologies* (pp. 44–88). Hershey, PA: IGI Global. doi:10.4018/978-1-4666-2979-0.ch004

McGaha, J. (2013). Implementation issues on a national electronic health record network. In I. Management Association (Ed.), User-driven healthcare: Concepts, methodologies, tools, and applications (pp. 1236-1251). Hershey, PA: IGI Global. doi:10.4018/978-1-4666-2770-3.ch062

McGinnes, S., & Burke, M. (2013). Hoping for the best: A qualitative study of information technology in primary care. In M. Cruz-Cunha, I. Miranda, & P. Gonçalves (Eds.), *Handbook of research on ICTs and management systems for improving efficiency in healthcare and social care* (pp. 1088–1108). Hershey, PA: IGI Global. doi:10.4018/978-1-4666-3990-4.ch057

Medhekar, A., Wong, H. Y., & Hall, J. (2014). Innovation in medical tourism service marketing: A case of India. In A. Goyal (Ed.), *Innovations in services marketing and management: Strategies for emerging economies* (pp. 49–66). Hershey, PA: IGI Global. doi:10.4018/978-1-4666-4671-1.ch003

Medhekar, A., Wong, H. Y., & Hall, J. (2014). Medical tourism: A conceptual framework for an innovation in global healthcare provision. In A. Goyal (Ed.), *Innovations in services marketing and management: Strategies for emerging economies* (pp. 148–169). Hershey, PA: IGI Global. doi:10.4018/978-1-4666-4671-1.ch009

Menciassi, A., & Laschi, C. (2014). Biorobotics. In I. Management Association (Ed.), Robotics: Concepts, methodologies, tools, and applications (pp. 1613-1643). Hershey, PA: IGI Global. doi:10.4018/978-1-4666-4607-0.ch079

Mendes, D., & Rodrigues, I. P. (2013). A semantic web pragmatic approach to develop clinical ontologies, and thus semantic interoperability, based in HL7 v2.xml messaging. In R. Martinho, R. Rijo, M. Cruz-Cunha, & J. Varajão (Eds.), *Information systems and technologies for enhancing health and social care* (pp. 205–214). Hershey, PA: IGI Global. doi:10.4018/978-1-4666-3667-5.ch014

Mendoza-González, R., Martin, M. V., & Rodríguez-Martínez, L. C. (2013). Identifying the essential design requirements for usable e-health communities in mobile devices. In I. Management Association (Ed.), User-driven healthcare: Concepts, methodologies, tools, and applications (pp. 533-552). Hershey, PA: IGI Global. doi:10.4018/978-1-4666-2770-3.ch027

Mettler, T. (2013). Transformation of the hospital supply chain: How to measure the maturity of supplier relationship management systems in hospitals? In J. Tan (Ed.), *Healthcare information technology innovation and sustainability: Frontiers and adoption* (pp. 180–192). Hershey, PA: IGI Global. doi:10.4018/978-1-4666-2797-0.ch011

Miesenberger, K., Nussbaum, G., & Ossmann, R. (2014). AsTeRICS: A framework for including sensor technology into AT solutions for people with motor disabilities. In G. Kouroupetroglou (Ed.), *Assistive technologies and computer access for motor disabilities* (pp. 154–179). Hershey, PA: IGI Global. doi:10.4018/978-1-4666-4438-0.ch006

Miller, K., & Sankaranarayanan, S. (2013). Applications of policy based agents in wireless body sensor mesh networks for patient health monitoring. In J. Rodrigues (Ed.), *Digital advances in medicine, e-health, and communication technologies* (pp. 85–101). Hershey, PA: IGI Global. doi:10.4018/978-1-4666-2794-9.ch005

Mohammadian, M., & Jentzsch, R. (2013). User and data classification for a secure and practical approach for patient-doctor profiling using an RFID framework in hospital. In S. Sarnikar, D. Bennett, & M. Gaynor (Eds.), *Cases on healthcare information technology for patient care management* (pp. 224–253). Hershey, PA: IGI Global. doi:10.4018/978-1-4666-2671-3.ch014

Monguet, J. M., Huerta, E., Fernández, J., Ferruzca, M., & Badillo, S. (2013). E-health business models prototyping by incremental design. In I. Management Association (Ed.), User-driven healthcare: Concepts, methodologies, tools, and applications (pp. 776-790). Hershey, PA: IGI Global. doi:10.4018/978-1-4666-2770-3.ch038

Montazemi, A. R., Pittaway, J. J., & Keshavjee, K. (2013). State of IS integration in the context of patient-centered care: A network analysis and research directions. In J. Tan (Ed.), *Healthcare information technology innovation and sustainability: Frontiers and adoption* (pp. 127–144). Hershey, PA: IGI Global. doi:10.4018/978-1-4666-2797-0.ch008

Mori, A. R., Contenti, M., & Verbicaro, R. (2013). Policies on telemedicine-enhanced hospital services: Prioritization criteria for the interventions at regional level. In V. Gulla, A. Mori, F. Gabbrielli, & P. Lanzafame (Eds.), *Telehealth networks for hospital services: New methodologies* (pp. 1–14). Hershey, PA: IGI Global. doi:10.4018/978-1-4666-2979-0.ch001

Morita, A. (2013). The quantitative EEG change in Parkinson's disease. In J. Wu (Ed.), *Biomedical engineering and cognitive neuroscience for healthcare: Interdisciplinary applications* (pp. 225–234). Hershey, PA: IGI Global. doi:10.4018/978-1-4666-2113-8.ch023

Moromugi, S., & Ishimatsu, T. (2013). A strength training machine with a dynamic resistance control function based on muscle activity level. In J. Wu (Ed.), *Technological advancements in biomedicine for healthcare applications* (pp. 102–110). Hershey, PA: IGI Global. doi:10.4018/978-1-4666-2196-1.ch011

Morrow, D., & Chin, J. (2013). Technology as a bridge between health care systems and older adults. In R. Zheng, R. Hill, & M. Gardner (Eds.), *Engaging older adults with modern technology: Internet use and information access needs* (pp. 59–79). Hershey, PA: IGI Global. doi:10.4018/978-1-4666-1966-1.ch004

Morrow, D., & Chin, J. (2013). Technology as a bridge between health care systems and older adults. In I. Management Association (Ed.), User-driven healthcare: Concepts, methodologies, tools, and applications (pp. 99-119). Hershey, PA: IGI Global. doi:10.4018/978-1-4666-2770-3.ch006

Mostafa, R., Hasan, G. M., Kabir, A. A., & Rahman, M. A. (2013). Proposed framework for the deployment of telemedicine centers in rural Bangladesh. In J. Rodrigues (Ed.), *Digital advances in medicine, e-health, and communication technologies* (pp. 254–270). Hershey, PA: IGI Global. doi:10.4018/978-1-4666-2794-9.ch014

Motoi, K., Ogawa, M., Yamakoshi, T., & Yamakoshi, K. (2013). Fusion physiological sensing system for healthcare. In J. Wu (Ed.), *Technological advancements in biomedicine for healthcare applications* (pp. 298–313). Hershey, PA: IGI Global. doi:10.4018/978-1-4666-2196-1.ch031

Motorny, S. P. (2013). Big information technology bet of a small community hospital. In S. Sarnikar, D. Bennett, & M. Gaynor (Eds.), *Cases on healthcare information technology for patient care management* (pp. 70–94). Hershey, PA: IGI Global. doi:10.4018/978-1-4666-2671-3.ch004

Moumtzoglou, A. (2013). Health 2.0 and medicine 2.0: Safety, ownership and privacy issues. In I. Management Association (Ed.), User-driven healthcare: Concepts, methodologies, tools, and applications (pp. 1508-1522). Hershey, PA: IGI Global. doi:10.4018/978-1-4666-2770-3.ch075

Moumtzoglou, A. (2013). Risk perception as a patient safety dimension. In A. Moumtzoglou & A. Kastania (Eds.), *E-health technologies and improving patient safety: Exploring organizational factors* (pp. 285–299). Hershey, PA: IGI Global. doi:10.4018/978-1-4666-2657-7.ch017

Msanjila, S. S. (2013). Emerging ICT challenges on provision of online HIV/AIDS advisory services. In M. Cruz-Cunha, I. Miranda, & P. Gonçalves (Eds.), *Handbook of research on ICTs for human-centered healthcare and social care services* (pp. 248–269). Hershey, PA: IGI Global. doi:10.4018/978-1-4666-3986-7.ch013

Müller, A. (2013). Improving the identification of medication names by increasing phonological awareness via a language-teaching computer game (medicina). In S. Arnab, I. Dunwell, & K. Debattista (Eds.), *Serious games for healthcare: Applications and implications* (pp. 283–295). Hershey, PA: IGI Global. doi:10.4018/978-1-4666-1903-6.ch014

Murakami, S., Kim, H., Tan, J. K., Ishikawa, S., & Aoki, T. (2013). The development of a quantitative method for the detection of periarticular osteoporosis using density features within ROIs from computed radiography images of the hand. In J. Wu (Ed.), *Technological advancements in biomedicine for healthcare applications* (pp. 55–67). Hershey, PA: IGI Global. doi:10.4018/978-1-4666-2196-1.ch007

Nadathur, S. G., & Warren, J. R. (2013). Formal-transfer in and out of stroke care units: An analysis using Bayesian networks. In J. Tan (Ed.), *Healthcare information technology innovation and sustainability: Frontiers and adoption* (pp. 193–207). Hershey, PA: IGI Global. doi:10.4018/978-1-4666-2797-0.ch012

Naidoo, V., & Naidoo, Y. (2014). Home telecare, medical implant, and mobile technology: Evolutions in geriatric care. In C. El Morr (Ed.), *Research perspectives on the role of informatics in health policy and management* (pp. 222–237). Hershey, PA: IGI Global. doi:10.4018/978-1-4666-4321-5.ch013

Nakagawa, S. (2013). Bone-conducted ultrasonic perception: An elucidation of perception mechanisms and the development of a novel hearing aid for the profoundly deaf. In J. Wu (Ed.), *Technological advancements in biomedicine for healthcare applications* (pp. 148–159). Hershey, PA: IGI Global. doi:10.4018/978-1-4666-2196-1.ch016

Nakai, M., & Niinomi, M. (2013). Recent progress in mechanically biocompatible titanium-based materials. In J. Wu (Ed.), *Technological advancements in biomedicine for healthcare applications* (pp. 206–212). Hershey, PA: IGI Global. doi:10.4018/978-1-4666-2196-1.ch022

Nakakuki, T., & Okada-Hatakeyama, M. (2013). Methods for the analysis of intracellular signal transduction systems. In J. Wu (Ed.), *Technological advancements in biomedicine for healthcare applications* (pp. 347–353). Hershey, PA: IGI Global. doi:10.4018/978-1-4666-2196-1.ch034

Nalin, M., Verga, M., Sanna, A., & Saranummi, N. (2013). Directions for ICT research in disease prevention. In M. Cruz-Cunha, I. Miranda, & P. Gonçalves (Eds.), *Handbook of research on ICTs for human-centered healthcare and social care services* (pp. 229–247). Hershey, PA: IGI Global. doi:10.4018/978-1-4666-3986-7.ch012

Nap, H. H., & Diaz-Orueta, U. (2013). Rehabilitation gaming. In S. Arnab, I. Dunwell, & K. Debattista (Eds.), *Serious games for healthcare: Applications and implications* (pp. 50–75). Hershey, PA: IGI Global. doi:10.4018/978-1-4666-1903-6.ch003

Narushima, T., & Ueda, K. (2013). Calcium phosphate coating on titanium by RF magnetron sputtering. In J. Wu (Ed.), *Technological advancements in biomedicine for healthcare applications* (pp. 223–233). Hershey, PA: IGI Global. doi:10.4018/978-1-4666-2196-1.ch024

Nava-Muñoz, S., & Morán, A. L. (2013). A review of notifications systems in elder care environments: Challenges and opportunities. In M. Cruz-Cunha, I. Miranda, & P. Gonçalves (Eds.), *Handbook of research on ICTs for human-centered healthcare and social care services* (pp. 407–429). Hershey, PA: IGI Global. doi:10.4018/978-1-4666-3986-7.ch022

Nganji, J. T., & Nggada, S. H. (2014). Adoption of blended learning technologies in selected secondary schools in Cameroon and Nigeria: Challenges in disability inclusion. In N. Ololube (Ed.), *Advancing technology and educational development through blended learning in emerging economies* (pp. 159–173). Hershey, PA: IGI Global. doi:10.4018/978-1-4666-4574-5.ch009

Nikolov, S., Vera, J., & Wolkenhauer, O. (2013). Bifurcation analysis of a model accounting for the 14-3-3s signalling compartmentalisation. In I. Management Association (Ed.), Bioinformatics: Concepts, methodologies, tools, and applications (pp. 851-859). Hershey, PA: IGI Global. doi:10.4018/978-1-4666-3604-0.ch046

Nishiguchi, H. (2013). Description of and applications for a motion analysis method for upper limbs. In J. Wu (Ed.), *Technological advancements in biomedicine for healthcare applications* (pp. 1–10). Hershey, PA: IGI Global. doi:10.4018/978-1-4666-2196-1.ch001

Nokata, M. (2013). Small medical robot. In J. Wu (Ed.), *Technological advancements in biomedicine for healthcare applications* (pp. 170–179). Hershey, PA: IGI Global. doi:10.4018/978-1-4666-2196-1.ch018

Noritsugu, T. (2013). Wearable power assist robot driven with pneumatic rubber artificial muscles. In J. Wu (Ed.), *Technological advancements in biomedicine for healthcare applications* (pp. 139–147). Hershey, PA: IGI Global. doi:10.4018/978-1-4666-2196-1.ch015

Noteboom, C. (2013). Physician interaction with EHR: The importance of stakeholder identification and change management. In S. Sarnikar, D. Bennett, & M. Gaynor (Eds.), *Cases on healthcare information technology for patient care management* (pp. 95–112). Hershey, PA: IGI Global. doi:10.4018/978-1-4666-2671-3.ch005

O'Hanlon, S. (2013). Avoiding adverse consequences of e-health. In A. Moumtzoglou & A. Kastania (Eds.), *E-health technologies and improving patient safety: Exploring organizational factors* (pp. 13–26). Hershey, PA: IGI Global. doi:10.4018/978-1-4666-2657-7.ch002

Ogawa, K., Nishio, S., Minato, T., & Ishiguro, H. (2013). Android robots as telepresence media. In J. Wu (Ed.), *Biomedical engineering and cognitive neuroscience for healthcare: Interdisciplinary applications* (pp. 54–63). Hershey, PA: IGI Global. doi:10.4018/978-1-4666-2113-8.ch006

Ohashi, M., Sakimura, N., Fujimoto, M., Hori, M., & Kurata, N. (2013). Technical perspective of authentication policy extension for the adaptive social services and e-health care management. In M. Cruz-Cunha, I. Miranda, & P. Gonçalves (Eds.), *Handbook of research on ICTs for human-centered healthcare and social care services* (pp. 719–726). Hershey, PA: IGI Global. doi:10.4018/978-1-4666-3986-7.ch037

Ohta, Y., & Uchida, M. (2013). Non-contact pulse monitoring using live imaging. In J. Wu (Ed.), *Technological advancements in biomedicine for healthcare applications* (pp. 240–246). Hershey, PA: IGI Global. doi:10.4018/978-1-4666-2196-1.ch026

Ohuchida, K., & Hashizume, M. (2013). Biomedical robotics for healthcare. In J. Wu (Ed.), *Technological advancements in biomedicine for healthcare applications* (pp. 200–205). Hershey, PA: IGI Global. doi:10.4018/978-1-4666-2196-1.ch021

Oikonomou, D., Moulianitis, V., Lekkas, D., & Koutsabasis, P. (2013). DSS for health emergency response: A contextual, user-centred approach. In R. Biswas (Ed.), *Clinical solutions and medical progress through user-driven healthcare* (pp. 51–69). Hershey, PA: IGI Global. doi:10.4018/978-1-4666-1876-3.ch006

Okamoto, S., Hirotomi, T., Aoki, K., & Hosomi, Y. (2013). Evaluation of walking motions with the aid of walkers using acceleration sensors. In J. Wu (Ed.), *Biomedical engineering and cognitive neuroscience for healthcare: Interdisciplinary applications* (pp. 346–354). Hershey, PA: IGI Global. doi:10.4018/978-1-4666-2113-8.ch036

Okamura, H. (2013). Rehabilitation of elderly people with dementia. In J. Wu (Ed.), *Biomedical engineering and cognitive neuroscience for healthcare: Interdisciplinary applications* (pp. 235–242). Hershey, PA: IGI Global. doi:10.4018/978-1-4666-2113-8.ch024

Olvera-Lobo, M., & Gutiérrez-Artacho, J. (2013). Searching health information in question-answering systems. In M. Cruz-Cunha, I. Miranda, & P. Gonçalves (Eds.), *Handbook of research on ICTs for human-centered healthcare and social care services* (pp. 474–490). Hershey, PA: IGI Global. doi:10.4018/978-1-4666-3986-7.ch025

Padovani, E., Orelli, R. L., Agnoletti, V., & Buccioli, M. (2013). Low cost and human-centered innovations in healthcare services: A case of excellence in Italy. In S. Saeed & C. Reddick (Eds.), *Human-centered system design for electronic governance* (pp. 239–252). Hershey, PA: IGI Global. doi:10.4018/978-1-4666-3640-8.ch014

Paninchukunnath, A. (2014). Healthcare services delivery in India: special reference to mother and child health. In A. Goyal (Ed.), *Innovations in services marketing and management: Strategies for emerging economies* (pp. 170–189). Hershey, PA: IGI Global. doi:10.4018/978-1-4666-4671-1.ch010

Paparountas, T., Nikolaidou-Katsaridou, M. N., Rustici, G., & Aidinis, V. (2013). Data mining and meta-analysis on DNA microarray data. In I. Management Association (Ed.), Bioinformatics: Concepts, methodologies, tools, and applications (pp. 1196-1236). Hershey, PA: IGI Global. doi:10.4018/978-1-4666-3604-0.ch062

Parentela, G., Mancini, P., Naccarella, F., Feng, Z., & Rinaldi, G. (2013). Telemedicine, the European space agency, and the support to the african population for infectious disease problems: Potentiality and perspectives for Asia countries and China. In V. Gulla, A. Mori, F. Gabbrielli, & P. Lanzafame (Eds.), *Telehealth networks for hospital services: New methodologies* (pp. 89–96). Hershey, PA: IGI Global. doi:10.4018/978-1-4666-2979-0.ch005

Paterson, G. I., MacDonald, J. M., & Mensink, N. N. (2014). The administrative policy quandary in Canada's health service organizations. In C. El Morr (Ed.), *Research perspectives on the role of informatics in health policy and management* (pp. 116–134). Hershey, PA: IGI Global. doi:10.4018/978-1-4666-4321-5.ch008

Penchovsky, R. (2013). Engineering gene control circuits with allosteric ribozymes in human cells as a medicine of the future. In I. Management Association (Ed.), Bioinformatics: Concepts, methodologies, tools, and applications (pp. 860-883). Hershey, PA: IGI Global. doi:10.4018/978-1-4666-3604-0.ch047

Pereira, O. R., Caldeira, J. M., & Rodrigues, J. J. (2013). An advanced and secure symbian-based mobile approach for body sensor networks interaction. In J. Rodrigues (Ed.), *Digital advances in medicine, e-health, and communication technologies* (pp. 33–48). Hershey, PA: IGI Global. doi:10.4018/978-1-4666-2794-9.ch002

Petkovic, M., & Ibraimi, L. (2013). Privacy and security in e-health applications. In I. Management Association (Ed.), User-driven healthcare: Concepts, methodologies, tools, and applications (pp. 1141-1166). Hershey, PA: IGI Global. doi:10.4018/978-1-4666-2770-3.ch058

Peyton, L., & Hu, J. (2013). Identity management and audit trail support for privacy protection in e-health networks. In I. Management Association (Ed.), User-driven healthcare: Concepts, methodologies, tools, and applications (pp. 1112-1125). Hershey, PA: IGI Global. doi:10.4018/978-1-4666-2770-3.ch056

Pham, D. V., Halgamuge, M. N., Nirmalathas, T., & Moran, B. (2013). A centralized real-time e-healthcare system for remote detection and prediction of epileptic seizures. In I. Management Association (Ed.), User-driven healthcare: Concepts, methodologies, tools, and applications (pp. 326-356). Hershey, PA: IGI Global. doi:10.4018/978-1-4666-2770-3.ch017

Phua, C., Roy, P. C., Aloulou, H., Biswas, J., Tolstikov, A., & Foo, V. S. … Xu, D. (2014). State-of-the-art assistive technology for people with dementia. In Assistive technologies: Concepts, methodologies, tools, and applications (pp. 1606-1625). Hershey, PA: IGI Global. doi:10.4018/978-1-4666-4422-9.ch085

Pino, A. (2014). Augmentative and alternative communication systems for the motor disabled. In G. Kouroupetroglou (Ed.), *Disability informatics and web accessibility for motor limitations* (pp. 105–152). Hershey, PA: IGI Global. doi:10.4018/978-1-4666-4442-7.ch004

Portela, F., Cabral, A., Abelha, A., Salazar, M., Quintas, C., Machado, J., ... Santos, M. F. (2013). Knowledge acquisition process for intelligent decision support in critical health care. In R. Martinho, R. Rijo, M. Cruz-Cunha, & J. Varajão (Eds.), *Information systems and technologies for enhancing health and social care* (pp. 55–68). Hershey, PA: IGI Global. doi:10.4018/978-1-4666-3667-5.ch004

Previtali, P. (2013). Grid technology for archive solutions in health care organizations. In A. Moumtzoglou & A. Kastania (Eds.), *E-health technologies and improving patient safety: Exploring organizational factors* (pp. 148–154). Hershey, PA: IGI Global. doi:10.4018/978-1-4666-2657-7.ch010

Purkayastha, S. (2013). Design and implementation of mobile-based technology in strengthening health information system: Aligning mhealth solutions to infrastructures. In I. Management Association (Ed.), User-driven healthcare: Concepts, methodologies, tools, and applications (pp. 689-713). Hershey, PA: IGI Global. doi:10.4018/978-1-4666-2770-3.ch034

Qi, G., & Wu, J. (2013). Functional role of the left ventral occipito-temporal cortex in reading. In J. Wu (Ed.), *Biomedical engineering and cognitive neuroscience for healthcare: Interdisciplinary applications* (pp. 192–200). Hershey, PA: IGI Global. doi:10.4018/978-1-4666-2113-8.ch020

Queirós, A., Alvarelhão, J., Silva, A. G., Teixeira, A., & Pacheco da Rocha, N. (2013). A conceptual framework for the design and development of AAL services. In M. Cruz-Cunha, I. Miranda, & P. Gonçalves (Eds.), *Handbook of research on ICTs for human-centered healthcare and social care services* (pp. 568–586). Hershey, PA: IGI Global. doi:10.4018/978-1-4666-3986-7.ch030

Ravka, N. (2014). Informatics and health services: The potential benefits and challenges of electronic health records and personal electronic health records in patient care, cost control, and health research – An overview. In C. El Morr (Ed.), *Research perspectives on the role of informatics in health policy and management* (pp. 89–114). Hershey, PA: IGI Global. doi:10.4018/978-1-4666-4321-5.ch007

Reibling, N., & Wendt, C. (2013). Regulating patients' access to healthcare services. In M. Merviö (Ed.), *Healthcare management and economics: Perspectives on public and private administration* (pp. 53–68). Hershey, PA: IGI Global. doi:10.4018/978-1-4666-3982-9.ch005

Reis, C. I., Freire, C. S., Fernández, J., & Monguet, J. M. (2013). Patient centered design: Challenges and lessons learned from working with health professionals and schizophrenic patients in e-therapy contexts. In R. Martinho, R. Rijo, M. Cruz-Cunha, & J. Varajão (Eds.), *Information systems and technologies for enhancing health and social care* (pp. 120–135). Hershey, PA: IGI Global. doi:10.4018/978-1-4666-3667-5.ch008

Remmers, H., & Hülsken-Giesler, M. (2013). e-Health technologies in home care nursing: Recent survey results and subsequent ethical issues. In I. Management Association (Ed.), User-driven healthcare: Concepts, methodologies, tools, and applications (pp. 396-420). Hershey, PA: IGI Global. doi:10.4018/978-1-4666-2770-3.ch020

Ricketts, M. (2014). Making health information personal: How anecdotes bring concepts to life. In S. Hai-Jew (Ed.), *Packaging digital information for enhanced learning and analysis: Data visualization, spatialization, and multidimensionality* (pp. 1–36). Hershey, PA: IGI Global. doi:10.4018/978-1-4666-4462-5.ch001

Rocha, Á. (2013). Evolution of information systems and technologies maturity in healthcare. In J. Tan (Ed.), *Healthcare information technology innovation and sustainability: Frontiers and adoption* (pp. 238–246). Hershey, PA: IGI Global. doi:10.4018/978-1-4666-2797-0.ch015

Rodríguez-Gómez, D., & Gairín, J. (2014). Communities of practice in the Catalan public administration: Promoting their improvement. In Y. Al-Bastaki & A. Shajera (Eds.), *Building a competitive public sector with knowledge management strategy* (pp. 383–402). Hershey, PA: IGI Global. doi:10.4018/978-1-4666-4434-2.ch018

Rodríguez-Solano, C., Lezcano, L., & Sicilia, M. (2013). Automated generation of SNOMED CT subsets from clinical guidelines. In R. Martinho, R. Rijo, M. Cruz-Cunha, & J. Varajão (Eds.), *Information systems and technologies for enhancing health and social care* (pp. 190–204). Hershey, PA: IGI Global. doi:10.4018/978-1-4666-3667-5.ch013

Rosu, S. M., & Dragoi, G. (2014). E-health sites development using open source software and OMT methodology as support for family doctors' activities: A Romanian case study. In M. Cruz-Cunha, F. Moreira, & J. Varajão (Eds.), *Handbook of research on enterprise 2.0: Technological, social, and organizational dimensions* (pp. 72–88). Hershey, PA: IGI Global. doi:10.4018/978-1-4666-4373-4.ch004

Roy, N., Das, S. K., & Julien, C. (2013). Resolving and mediating ambiguous contexts in pervasive environments. In I. Management Association (Ed.), User-driven healthcare: Concepts, methodologies, tools, and applications (pp. 630-654). Hershey, PA: IGI Global. doi:10.4018/978-1-4666-2770-3.ch031

Russo, M. R. (2014). Emergency management professional development: Linking information communication technology and social communication skills to enhance a sense of community and social justice in the 21st century. In I. Management Association (Ed.), Crisis management: Concepts, methodologies, tools and applications (pp. 651-665). Hershey, PA: IGI Global. doi:10.4018/978-1-4666-4707-7.ch031

Sabone, M. B., Mogobe, K. D., & Sabone, T. G. (2013). ICTS and their role in health promotion: A preliminary situation analysis in selected botswana rural communities. In I. Management Association (Ed.), User-driven healthcare: Concepts, methodologies, tools, and applications (pp. 211-224). Hershey, PA: IGI Global. doi:10.4018/978-1-4666-2770-3.ch012

Saha, P. (2014). Systemic enterprise architecture as future: Tackling complexity in governments in the cusp of change. In P. Saha (Ed.), *A systemic perspective to managing complexity with enterprise architecture* (pp. 1–70). Hershey, PA: IGI Global. doi:10.4018/978-1-4666-4518-9.ch001

Saijo, Y. (2013). Biomedical application of multimodal ultrasound microscope. In J. Wu (Ed.), *Technological advancements in biomedicine for healthcare applications* (pp. 27–35). Hershey, PA: IGI Global. doi:10.4018/978-1-4666-2196-1.ch004

Santos, M., Bastião, L., Costa, C., Silva, A., & Rocha, N. (2013). Clinical data mining in small hospital PACS: Contributions for radiology department improvement. In R. Martinho, R. Rijo, M. Cruz-Cunha, & J. Varajão (Eds.), *Information systems and technologies for enhancing health and social care* (pp. 236–251). Hershey, PA: IGI Global. doi:10.4018/978-1-4666-3667-5.ch016

Santos, M. F., Portela, F., Miranda, M., Machado, J., Abelha, A., Silva, Á., & Rua, F. (2013). Grid data mining strategies for outcome prediction in distributed intensive care units. In R. Martinho, R. Rijo, M. Cruz-Cunha, & J. Varajão (Eds.), *Information systems and technologies for enhancing health and social care* (pp. 87–101). Hershey, PA: IGI Global. doi:10.4018/978-1-4666-3667-5.ch006

Santos, R. J., Bernardino, J., & Vieira, M. (2013). A hypotension surveillance and prediction system for critical care. In M. Cruz-Cunha, I. Miranda, & P. Gonçalves (Eds.), *Handbook of research on ICTs and management systems for improving efficiency in healthcare and social care* (pp. 341–355). Hershey, PA: IGI Global. doi:10.4018/978-1-4666-3990-4.ch017

Sanz, P. R., Mezcua, B. R., & Pena, J. M. (2013). ICTs for orientation and mobility for blind people: A state of the art. In M. Cruz-Cunha, I. Miranda, & P. Gonçalves (Eds.), *Handbook of research on ICTs for human-centered healthcare and social care services* (pp. 646–669). Hershey, PA: IGI Global. doi:10.4018/978-1-4666-3986-7.ch034

Sarabdeen, J. (2013). Legal issues in e-healthcare systems. In I. Management Association (Ed.), User-driven healthcare: Concepts, methodologies, tools, and applications (pp. 1194-1219). Hershey, PA: IGI Global. doi:10.4018/978-1-4666-2770-3.ch060

Sarbadhikari, S. N. (2013). Unlearning and relearning in online health education. In I. Management Association (Ed.), User-driven healthcare: Concepts, methodologies, tools, and applications (pp. 1348-1363). Hershey, PA: IGI Global. doi:10.4018/978-1-4666-2770-3.ch067

Sasayama, T., Hamada, S., & Kobayashi, T. (2013). Application of prewhitening beamformer with linear constraints for correlated EEG signal source estimation. In J. Wu (Ed.), *Biomedical engineering and cognitive neuroscience for healthcare: Interdisciplinary applications* (pp. 243–254). Hershey, PA: IGI Global. doi:10.4018/978-1-4666-2113-8.ch025

Sato, T., & Minato, K. (2013). Differences in analysis methods of the human uncinate fasciculus using diffusion tensor MRI. In J. Wu (Ed.), *Biomedical engineering and cognitive neuroscience for healthcare: Interdisciplinary applications* (pp. 162–170). Hershey, PA: IGI Global. doi:10.4018/978-1-4666-2113-8.ch017

Satoh, J. (2013). Molecular network analysis of target RNAs and interacting proteins of TDP-43, a causative gene for the neurodegenerative diseases ALS/FTLD. In I. Management Association (Ed.), Bioinformatics: Concepts, methodologies, tools, and applications (pp. 964-985). Hershey, PA: IGI Global. doi:10.4018/978-1-4666-3604-0.ch052

Satoh, J. (2013). Molecular network analysis of target RNAs and interacting proteins of TDP-43, a causative gene for the neurodegenerative diseases ALS/FTLD. In J. Wu (Ed.), *Technological advancements in biomedicine for healthcare applications* (pp. 314–335). Hershey, PA: IGI Global. doi:10.4018/978-1-4666-2196-1.ch032

Schafer, S. B. (2013). Fostering psychological coherence: With ICTs. In M. Cruz-Cunha, I. Miranda, & P. Gonçalves (Eds.), *Handbook of research on ICTs for human-centered healthcare and social care services* (pp. 29–47). Hershey, PA: IGI Global. doi:10.4018/978-1-4666-3986-7.ch002

Schmeida, M., & McNeal, R. (2013). Bridging the inequality gap to accessing medicare and medicaid information online: An empirical analysis of e-government success 2002 through 2010. In J. Gil-Garcia (Ed.), *E-government success around the world: Cases, empirical studies, and practical recommendations* (pp. 60–78). Hershey, PA: IGI Global. doi:10.4018/978-1-4666-4173-0.ch004

Scholl, J. C., & Olaniran, B. A. (2013). ICT use and multidisciplinary healthcare teams. In M. Cruz-Cunha, I. Miranda, & P. Gonçalves (Eds.), *Handbook of research on ICTs for human-centered healthcare and social care services* (pp. 627–645). Hershey, PA: IGI Global. doi:10.4018/978-1-4666-3986-7.ch033

Serenko, N. (2013). The impact of genetic testing and genetic information on ethical, legal and social issues in North America: The framework. In I. Management Association (Ed.), Bioinformatics: Concepts, methodologies, tools, and applications (pp. 1317-1333). Hershey, PA: IGI Global. doi:10.4018/978-1-4666-3604-0.ch067

Serrano, M., Elmisery, A., Foghlú, M. Ó., Donnelly, W., Storni, C., & Fernström, M. (2013). Pervasive computing support in the transition towards personalised health systems. In J. Rodrigues (Ed.), *Digital advances in medicine, e-health, and communication technologies* (pp. 49–64). Hershey, PA: IGI Global. doi:10.4018/978-1-4666-2794-9.ch003

Shaw, V., & Braa, J. (2013). "Developed in the south": An evolutionary and prototyping approach to developing scalable and sustainable health information systems. In I. Management Association (Ed.), User-driven healthcare: Concepts, methodologies, tools, and applications (pp. 583-607). Hershey, PA: IGI Global. doi:10.4018/978-1-4666-2770-3.ch029

Shi, J., Upadhyaya, S., & Erdem, E. (2013). Health information exchange for improving the efficiency and quality of healthcare delivery. In I. Management Association (Ed.), User-driven healthcare: Concepts, methodologies, tools, and applications (pp. 714-736). Hershey, PA: IGI Global. doi:10.4018/978-1-4666-2770-3.ch035

Shibata, T. (2013). A human-like cognitive computer based on a psychologically inspired VLSI brain model. In J. Wu (Ed.), *Technological advancements in biomedicine for healthcare applications* (pp. 247–266). Hershey, PA: IGI Global. doi:10.4018/978-1-4666-2196-1.ch027

Shimada, S. (2013). Self-body recognition and its impairment. In J. Wu (Ed.), *Biomedical engineering and cognitive neuroscience for healthcare: Interdisciplinary applications* (pp. 156–161). Hershey, PA: IGI Global. doi:10.4018/978-1-4666-2113-8.ch016

Shimogonya, Y., Ishikawa, T., Yamaguchi, T., Kumamaru, H., & Itoh, K. (2013). Computational study of the hemodynamics of cerebral aneurysm initiation. In J. Wu (Ed.), *Technological advancements in biomedicine for healthcare applications* (pp. 267–277). Hershey, PA: IGI Global. doi:10.4018/978-1-4666-2196-1.ch028

Shimonomura, K. (2013). A neuromorphic robot vision system to predict the response of visual neurons. In J. Wu (Ed.), *Technological advancements in biomedicine for healthcare applications* (pp. 193–199). Hershey, PA: IGI Global. doi:10.4018/978-1-4666-2196-1.ch020

Shrestha, S. (2013). Clinical decision support system for diabetes prevention: An illustrative case. In S. Sarnikar, D. Bennett, & M. Gaynor (Eds.), *Cases on healthcare information technology for patient care management* (pp. 308–329). Hershey, PA: IGI Global. doi:10.4018/978-1-4666-2671-3.ch017

Siddiqui, Z. S., & Jonas-Dwyer, D. R. (2013). Mobile learning in health professions education: A systematic review. In J. Keengwe (Ed.), *Pedagogical applications and social effects of mobile technology integration* (pp. 193–205). Hershey, PA: IGI Global. doi:10.4018/978-1-4666-2985-1.ch011

Silvana de Rosa, A., Fino, E., & Bocci, E. (2014). Addressing healthcare on-line demand and supply relating to mental illness: Knowledge sharing about psychiatry and psychoanalysis through social networks in Italy and France. In A. Kapoor & C. Kulshrestha (Eds.), *Dynamics of competitive advantage and consumer perception in social marketing* (pp. 16–55). Hershey, PA: IGI Global. doi:10.4018/978-1-4666-4430-4.ch002

Siqueira, S. R., Rocha, E. C., & Nery, M. S. (2013). Brazilian occupational therapy perspective about digital games as an inclusive resource to disabled people in schools. In I. Management Association (Ed.), User-driven healthcare: Concepts, methodologies, tools, and applications (pp. 918-937). Hershey, PA: IGI Global. doi:10.4018/978-1-4666-2770-3.ch046

Sliedrecht, S., & Kotzé, E. (2013). Patients with a spinal cord injury inform and co-construct services at a spinal cord rehabilitation unit. In I. Management Association (Ed.), User-driven healthcare: Concepts, methodologies, tools, and applications (pp. 1054-1072). Hershey, PA: IGI Global. doi:10.4018/978-1-4666-2770-3.ch053

Smedberg, Å. (2013). E-health communities for learning healthy habits: How to consider quality and usability. In I. Management Association (Ed.), User-driven healthcare: Concepts, methodologies, tools, and applications (pp. 310-325). Hershey, PA: IGI Global. doi:10.4018/978-1-4666-2770-3.ch016

Smedberg, Å., & Sandmark, H. (2013). Dynamic stress management: Self-help through holistic system design. In I. Management Association (Ed.), User-driven healthcare: Concepts, methodologies, tools, and applications (pp. 1469-1486). Hershey, PA: IGI Global. doi:10.4018/978-1-4666-2770-3.ch073

Sobol, M., & Prater, E. (2013). Adoption, usage and efficiency: Benchmarking healthcare IT in private practices. In J. Tan (Ed.), *Healthcare information technology innovation and sustainability: Frontiers and adoption* (pp. 145–159). Hershey, PA: IGI Global. doi:10.4018/978-1-4666-2797-0.ch009

Sobrinho, Á. A., Dias da Silva, L., Melo de Medeiros, L., & Pinheiro, M. E. (2013). A mobile assistant to aid early detection of chronic kidney disease. In R. Martinho, R. Rijo, M. Cruz-Cunha, & J. Varajão (Eds.), *Information systems and technologies for enhancing health and social care* (pp. 309–323). Hershey, PA: IGI Global. doi:10.4018/978-1-4666-3667-5.ch020

Soomlek, C., & Benedicenti, L. (2013). Agent-based wellness indicator. In V. Gulla, A. Mori, F. Gabbrielli, & P. Lanzafame (Eds.), *Telehealth networks for hospital services: New methodologies* (pp. 300–330). Hershey, PA: IGI Global. doi:10.4018/978-1-4666-2979-0.ch020

Spadaro, L., Timpano, F., Marino, S., & Bramanti, P. (2013). Telemedicine and Alzheimer disease: ICT-based services for people with Alzheimer disease and their caregivers. In V. Gulla, A. Mori, F. Gabbrielli, & P. Lanzafame (Eds.), *Telehealth networks for hospital services: New methodologies* (pp. 191–206). Hershey, PA: IGI Global. doi:10.4018/978-1-4666-2979-0.ch013

Springer, J. A., Beever, J., Morar, N., Sprague, J. E., & Kane, M. D. (2013). Ethics, privacy, and the future of genetic information in healthcare information assurance and security. In I. Management Association (Ed.), Bioinformatics: Concepts, methodologies, tools, and applications (pp. 1405-1423). Hershey, PA: IGI Global. doi:10.4018/978-1-4666-3604-0.ch072

Stachura, M. E., Wood, J., Angjellari-Dajci, F., Grayson, J., Astapova, E. V., Tung, H., . . . Lawless, W. (2013). Representing organizational conservation of information: A review of telemedicine and e-health in Georgia. In I. Management Association (Ed.), User-driven healthcare: Concepts, methodologies, tools, and applications (pp. 1220-1235). Hershey, PA: IGI Global. doi:10.4018/978-1-4666-2770-3.ch061

Stefaniak, J. E. (2013). Resuscitating team roles within wayburn health system. In A. Ritzhaupt & S. Kumar (Eds.), *Cases on educational technology implementation for facilitating learning* (pp. 130–145). Hershey, PA: IGI Global. doi:10.4018/978-1-4666-3676-7.ch008

Sugiura, M. (2013). A cognitive neuroscience approach to self and mental health. In J. Wu (Ed.), *Biomedical engineering and cognitive neuroscience for healthcare: Interdisciplinary applications* (pp. 1–10). Hershey, PA: IGI Global. doi:10.4018/978-1-4666-2113-8.ch001

Supnithi, T., Buranarach, M., Thatphithakkul, N., Junsirimongkol, B., Wongrochananan, S., Kulnawan, N., & Jiamjarasrangsi, W. (2014). A self-management service framework to support chronic disease patients' self-management. In M. Kosaka & K. Shirahada (Eds.), *Progressive trends in knowledge and system-based science for service innovation* (pp. 425–450). Hershey, PA: IGI Global. doi:10.4018/978-1-4666-4663-6.ch023

Takahashi, K., & Watanabe, K. (2013). Crossmodal interactions in visual competition. In J. Wu (Ed.), *Biomedical engineering and cognitive neuroscience for healthcare: Interdisciplinary applications* (pp. 64–72). Hershey, PA: IGI Global. doi:10.4018/978-1-4666-2113-8.ch007

Tamiya, T., Kawanishi, M., Miyake, K., Kawai, N., & Guo, S. (2013). Neurosurgical operations using navigation microscope integration system. In J. Wu (Ed.), *Technological advancements in biomedicine for healthcare applications* (pp. 128–138). Hershey, PA: IGI Global. doi:10.4018/978-1-4666-2196-1.ch014

Tan, R., Wang, S., Jiang, Y., Ishida, K., & Fujie, M. G. (2013). Motion control of an omni-directional walker for walking support. In J. Wu (Ed.), *Biomedical engineering and cognitive neuroscience for healthcare: Interdisciplinary applications* (pp. 20–28). Hershey, PA: IGI Global. doi:10.4018/978-1-4666-2113-8.ch003

Tanaka, H., & Furutani, M. (2013). Sleep management promotes healthy lifestyle, mental health, QOL, and a healthy brain. In J. Wu (Ed.), *Biomedical engineering and cognitive neuroscience for healthcare: Interdisciplinary applications* (pp. 211–224). Hershey, PA: IGI Global. doi:10.4018/978-1-4666-2113-8.ch022

Tang, C., & Carpendale, S. (2013). Human-centered design for health information technology: A qualitative approach. In I. Management Association (Ed.), User-driven healthcare: Concepts, methodologies, tools, and applications (pp. 158-179). Hershey, PA: IGI Global. doi:10.4018/978-1-4666-2770-3.ch009

Tang, X., Gao, Y., Yang, W., Zhang, M., & Wu, J. (2013). Audiovisual integration of natural auditory and visual stimuli in the real-world situation. In J. Wu (Ed.), *Biomedical engineering and cognitive neuroscience for healthcare: Interdisciplinary applications* (pp. 337–344). Hershey, PA: IGI Global. doi:10.4018/978-1-4666-2113-8.ch035

Targowski, A. (2013). Well-being, wisdom, health, and IT: From the big-picture to the small-picture. In M. Cruz-Cunha, I. Miranda, & P. Gonçalves (Eds.), *Handbook of research on ICTs for human-centered healthcare and social care services* (pp. 1–28). Hershey, PA: IGI Global. doi:10.4018/978-1-4666-3986-7.ch001

Tayabali, S., & Martin, C. M. (2013). The need to transform the core values of medical care and health organizations. In R. Biswas (Ed.), *Clinical solutions and medical progress through user-driven healthcare* (pp. 85–92). Hershey, PA: IGI Global. doi:10.4018/978-1-4666-1876-3.ch009

Taylor, B. W. (2014). Decision-making and decision support in acute care. In C. El Morr (Ed.), *Research perspectives on the role of informatics in health policy and management* (pp. 1–18). Hershey, PA: IGI Global. doi:10.4018/978-1-4666-4321-5.ch001

Teixeira, C., Pinto, J. S., Ferreira, F., Oliveira, A., Teixeira, A., & Pereira, C. (2013). Cloud computing enhanced service development architecture for the living usability lab. In R. Martinho, R. Rijo, M. Cruz-Cunha, & J. Varajão (Eds.), *Information systems and technologies for enhancing health and social care* (pp. 33–53). Hershey, PA: IGI Global. doi:10.4018/978-1-4666-3667-5.ch003

Teixeira, L., Saavedra, V., Ferreira, C., & Santos, B. S. (2013). The role of ICTs in the management of rare chronic diseases: The case of hemophilia. In M. Cruz-Cunha, I. Miranda, & P. Gonçalves (Eds.), *Handbook of research on ICTs and management systems for improving efficiency in healthcare and social care* (pp. 635–649). Hershey, PA: IGI Global. doi:10.4018/978-1-4666-3990-4.ch033

Teoh, S. Y., Singh, M., & Chong, J. (2013). An overview of e-health development in Australia. In I. Management Association (Ed.), User-driven healthcare: Concepts, methodologies, tools, and applications (pp. 901-917). Hershey, PA: IGI Global. doi:10.4018/978-1-4666-2770-3.ch045

Tiwari, S., & Srivastava, R. (2014). Research and developments in medical image reconstruction methods and its applications. In R. Srivastava, S. Singh, & K. Shukla (Eds.), *Research developments in computer vision and image processing: Methodologies and applications* (pp. 274–312). Hershey, PA: IGI Global. doi:10.4018/978-1-4666-4558-5.ch014

Tobolcea, I. (2013). The psychosocial impact of ICT efficiency on speech disorders-treatment. In M. Cruz-Cunha, I. Miranda, & P. Gonçalves (Eds.), *Handbook of research on ICTs for human-centered healthcare and social care services* (pp. 70–92). Hershey, PA: IGI Global. doi:10.4018/978-1-4666-3986-7.ch004

Toda, T., Chen, P., Ozaki, S., Fujita, K., & Ideguchi, N. (2013). A simple web-based image database system for facilitating medical care in dermatological clinics. In I. Management Association (Ed.), User-driven healthcare: Concepts, methodologies, tools, and applications (pp. 502-513). Hershey, PA: IGI Global. doi:10.4018/978-1-4666-2770-3.ch025

Toda, T., Chen, P., Ozaki, S., Fujita, K., & Ideguchi, N. (2013). A simple web-based image database system for facilitating medical care in dermatological clinics. In J. Wu (Ed.), *Technological advancements in biomedicine for healthcare applications* (pp. 385–397). Hershey, PA: IGI Global. doi:10.4018/978-1-4666-2196-1.ch038

Trudeau, S. (2013). CoRDS registry: An HIT case study concerning setup and maintenance of a disease registry. In S. Sarnikar, D. Bennett, & M. Gaynor (Eds.), *Cases on healthcare information technology for patient care management* (pp. 197–207). Hershey, PA: IGI Global. doi:10.4018/978-1-4666-2671-3.ch012

Tseng, R., & Yi-Luen Do, E. (2013). The role of information and computer technology for children with autism spectrum disorder and the facial expression wonderland (FEW). In A. Gangopadhyay (Ed.), *Methods, models, and computation for medical informatics* (pp. 98–116). Hershey, PA: IGI Global. doi:10.4018/978-1-4666-2653-9.ch006

Uchitomi, H., Suzuki, K., Nishi, T., Hove, M. J., Miyake, Y., Orimo, S., & Wada, Y. (2013). Gait rhythm of Parkinson's disease patients and an interpersonal synchrony emulation system based on cooperative gait. In J. Wu (Ed.), *Biomedical engineering and cognitive neuroscience for healthcare: Interdisciplinary applications* (pp. 38–53). Hershey, PA: IGI Global. doi:10.4018/978-1-4666-2113-8.ch005

Usher, W., & San Too, L. (2013). E-health knowledge management by australian university students. In I. Management Association (Ed.), User-driven healthcare: Concepts, methodologies, tools, and applications (pp. 938-953). Hershey, PA: IGI Global. doi:10.4018/978-1-4666-2770-3.ch047

Van Genderen, E. (2014). Intensive care. In V. Jham & S. Puri (Eds.), *Cases on consumer-centric marketing management* (pp. 53–67). Hershey, PA: IGI Global. doi:10.4018/978-1-4666-4357-4.ch006

Van Leuven, N., Newton, D., Leuenberger, D. Z., & Esteves, T. (2014). Reaching citizen 2.0: How government uses social media to send public messages during times of calm and times of crisis. In I. Management Association (Ed.), Crisis management: Concepts, methodologies, tools and applications (pp. 839-857). Hershey, PA: IGI Global. doi:10.4018/978-1-4666-4707-7.ch041

Vasudevan, V., & Rao, H. (2013). E-discovery and health care IT: An investigation. In I. Management Association (Ed.), User-driven healthcare: Concepts, methodologies, tools, and applications (pp. 1622-1635). Hershey, PA: IGI Global. doi:10.4018/978-1-4666-2770-3.ch080

Vat, K. H. (2013). Conceiving community knowledge records as e-governance concerns in wired healthcare provision. In I. Management Association (Ed.), User-driven healthcare: Concepts, methodologies, tools, and applications (pp. 1093-1111). Hershey, PA: IGI Global. doi:10.4018/978-1-4666-2770-3.ch055

Venkatasubramanian, K. K., Nabar, S., Gupta, S. K., & Poovendran, R. (2013). Cyber physical security solutions for pervasive health monitoring systems. In I. Management Association (Ed.), User-driven healthcare: Concepts, methodologies, tools, and applications (pp. 447-465). Hershey, PA: IGI Global. doi:10.4018/978-1-4666-2770-3.ch022

Victan, H. (2013). Emerging trends in user-driven healthcare: Negotiating disclosure in online health community organizations. In I. Management Association (Ed.), User-driven healthcare: Concepts, methodologies, tools, and applications (pp. 1589-1606). Hershey, PA: IGI Global. doi:10.4018/978-1-4666-2770-3.ch078

Vidal, B., Pereira, J. M., & Santos, G. (2013). SimBody: An interactive simulator for health education. In S. Arnab, I. Dunwell, & K. Debattista (Eds.), *Serious games for healthcare: Applications and implications* (pp. 265–282). Hershey, PA: IGI Global. doi:10.4018/978-1-4666-1903-6.ch013

Vivekananda-Schmidt, P. (2013). Ethics in the design of serious games for healthcare and medicine. In S. Arnab, I. Dunwell, & K. Debattista (Eds.), *Serious games for healthcare: Applications and implications* (pp. 91–106). Hershey, PA: IGI Global. doi:10.4018/978-1-4666-1903-6.ch005

Wahbeh, A. (2013). Application of handheld computing and mobile phones in diabetes self-care. In S. Sarnikar, D. Bennett, & M. Gaynor (Eds.), *Cases on healthcare information technology for patient care management* (pp. 254–275). Hershey, PA: IGI Global. doi:10.4018/978-1-4666-2671-3.ch015

Waidyanatha, N., & Dekker, S. (2013). The RTBP – Collective intelligence driving health for the user. In R. Biswas (Ed.), *Clinical solutions and medical progress through user-driven healthcare* (pp. 70–78). Hershey, PA: IGI Global. doi:10.4018/978-1-4666-1876-3.ch007

Waidyanatha, N., Dubrawski, A. M. G., & Gow, G. (2013). Affordable system for rapid detection and mitigation of emerging diseases. In J. Rodrigues (Ed.), *Digital advances in medicine, e-health, and communication technologies* (pp. 271–288). Hershey, PA: IGI Global. doi:10.4018/978-1-4666-2794-9.ch015

Walker, D. (2013). How would a ban on prescriber-identifying information impact pharmaceutical marketing? In M. Merviö (Ed.), *Healthcare management and economics: Perspectives on public and private administration* (pp. 141–153). Hershey, PA: IGI Global. doi:10.4018/978-1-4666-3982-9.ch011

Wang, B., Yan, T., & Wu, J. (2013). Neuronal function in the cortical face perception network. In J. Wu (Ed.), *Biomedical engineering and cognitive neuroscience for healthcare: Interdisciplinary applications* (pp. 171–182). Hershey, PA: IGI Global. doi:10.4018/978-1-4666-2113-8.ch018

Wang, Y., & Wang, Q. (2013). Evaluating the IEEE 802.15.6 2.4GHz WBAN proposal on medical multi-parameter monitoring under WiFi/bluetooth interference. In J. Rodrigues (Ed.), *Digital advances in medicine, e-health, and communication technologies* (pp. 312–325). Hershey, PA: IGI Global. doi:10.4018/978-1-4666-2794-9.ch018

Watanabe, T., & Miura, N. (2013). Functional electrical stimulation (FES) control for restoration and rehabilitation of motor function. In J. Wu (Ed.), *Technological advancements in biomedicine for healthcare applications* (pp. 80–93). Hershey, PA: IGI Global. doi:10.4018/978-1-4666-2196-1.ch009

Watanabe, Y., Tanaka, H., & Hirata, K. (2013). Evaluation of cognitive function in migraine patients: A study using event-related potentials. In J. Wu (Ed.), *Biomedical engineering and cognitive neuroscience for healthcare: Interdisciplinary applications* (pp. 303–310). Hershey, PA: IGI Global. doi:10.4018/978-1-4666-2113-8.ch031

Watfa, M. K., Kaur, M., & Daruwala, R. F. (2013). RFID applications in e-healthcare. In I. Management Association (Ed.), User-driven healthcare: Concepts, methodologies, tools, and applications (pp. 259-287). Hershey, PA: IGI Global. doi:10.4018/978-1-4666-2770-3.ch014

Wesorick, B. (2013). Essential steps for successful implementation of the EHR to achieve sustainable, safe, quality care. In A. Moumtzoglou & A. Kastania (Eds.), *E-health technologies and improving patient safety: Exploring organizational factors* (pp. 27–55). Hershey, PA: IGI Global. doi:10.4018/978-1-4666-2657-7.ch003

Whitaker, R. (2013). Securing health-effective medicine in practice: A critical perspective on user-driven healthcare. In R. Biswas (Ed.), *Clinical solutions and medical progress through user-driven healthcare* (pp. 35–50). Hershey, PA: IGI Global. doi:10.4018/978-1-4666-1876-3.ch005

Wickramasinghe, N., Troshani, I., Hill, S. R., Hague, W., & Goldberg, S. (2013). A transaction cost assessment of a pervasive technology solution for gestational diabetes. In J. Tan (Ed.), *Healthcare information technology innovation and sustainability: Frontiers and adoption* (pp. 109–126). Hershey, PA: IGI Global. doi:10.4018/978-1-4666-2797-0.ch007

Wilkowska, W., & Ziefle, M. (2013). User diversity as a challenge for the integration of medical technology into future smart home environments. In I. Management Association (Ed.), User-driven healthcare: Concepts, methodologies, tools, and applications (pp. 553-582). Hershey, PA: IGI Global. doi:10.4018/978-1-4666-2770-3.ch028

Willis, E., Wang, Y., & Rodgers, S. (2013). Online health communities and health literacy: Applying a framework for understanding domains of health literacy. In I. Management Association (Ed.), User-driven healthcare: Concepts, methodologies, tools, and applications (pp. 180-196). Hershey, PA: IGI Global. doi:10.4018/978-1-4666-2770-3.ch010

Wu, Q., Li, C., Takahashi, S., & Wu, J. (2013). Visual-tactile bottom-up and top-down attention. In J. Wu (Ed.), *Biomedical engineering and cognitive neuroscience for healthcare: Interdisciplinary applications* (pp. 183–191). Hershey, PA: IGI Global. doi:10.4018/978-1-4666-2113-8.ch019

Yamaguchi, S., Onoda, K., & Abe, S. (2013). Feedback-related negativity and its clinical implications. In J. Wu (Ed.), *Biomedical engineering and cognitive neuroscience for healthcare: Interdisciplinary applications* (pp. 283–292). Hershey, PA: IGI Global. doi:10.4018/978-1-4666-2113-8.ch029

Yan, B., Lei, Y., Tong, L., & Chen, K. (2013). Functional neuroimaging of acupuncture: A systematic review. In J. Wu (Ed.), *Biomedical engineering and cognitive neuroscience for healthcare: Interdisciplinary applications* (pp. 142–155). Hershey, PA: IGI Global. doi:10.4018/978-1-4666-2113-8.ch015

Yang, J. (2014). Towards healthy public policy: GIS and food systems analysis. In C. El Morr (Ed.), *Research perspectives on the role of informatics in health policy and management* (pp. 135–152). Hershey, PA: IGI Global. doi:10.4018/978-1-4666-4321-5.ch009

Yang, J., Li, Q., Gao, Y., & Wu, J. (2013). Temporal dependency of multisensory audiovisual integration. In J. Wu (Ed.), *Biomedical engineering and cognitive neuroscience for healthcare: Interdisciplinary applications* (pp. 320–326). Hershey, PA: IGI Global. doi:10.4018/978-1-4666-2113-8.ch033

Yang, J. J., Liu, J. F., Kurokawa, T., Kitamura, N., Yasuda, K., & Gong, J. P. (2013). Tough double-network hydrogels as scaffolds for tissue engineering: Cell behavior in vitro and in vivo test. In J. Wu (Ed.), *Technological advancements in biomedicine for healthcare applications* (pp. 213–222). Hershey, PA: IGI Global. doi:10.4018/978-1-4666-2196-1.ch023

Yang, W., Gao, Y., & Wu, J. (2013). Effects of selective and divided attention on audiovisual interaction. In J. Wu (Ed.), *Biomedical engineering and cognitive neuroscience for healthcare: Interdisciplinary applications* (pp. 311–319). Hershey, PA: IGI Global. doi:10.4018/978-1-4666-2113-8.ch032

Yano, Y. (2013). An EMG control system for an ultrasonic motor using a PSoC microcomputer. In J. Wu (Ed.), *Technological advancements in biomedicine for healthcare applications* (pp. 11–17). Hershey, PA: IGI Global. doi:10.4018/978-1-4666-2196-1.ch002

Yap, K. Y. (2013). The evolving role of pharmacoinformatics in targeting drug-related problems in clinical oncology practice. In I. Management Association (Ed.), User-driven healthcare: Concepts, methodologies, tools, and applications (pp. 1541-1588). Hershey, PA: IGI Global. doi:10.4018/978-1-4666-2770-3.ch077

Yokoi, H., Kato, R., Mori, T., Yamamura, O., & Kubota, M. (2013). Functional electrical stimulation based on interference-driven PWM signals for neuro-rehabilitation. In J. Wu (Ed.), *Technological advancements in biomedicine for healthcare applications* (pp. 180–192). Hershey, PA: IGI Global. doi:10.4018/978-1-4666-2196-1.ch019

York, A. M., & Nordengren, F. R. (2013). E-learning and web 2.0 case study: The role of gender in contemporary models of health care leadership. In H. Yang & S. Wang (Eds.), *Cases on formal and informal e-learning environments: Opportunities and practices* (pp. 292–313). Hershey, PA: IGI Global. doi:10.4018/978-1-4666-1930-2.ch016

Yu, W. D., & Bhagwat, R. (2013). Modeling emergency and telemedicine health support system: A service oriented architecture approach using cloud computing. In J. Rodrigues (Ed.), *Digital advances in medicine, e-health, and communication technologies* (pp. 187–213). Hershey, PA: IGI Global. doi:10.4018/978-1-4666-2794-9.ch011

Yu, Y., Yang, J., & Wu, J. (2013). Cognitive functions and neuronal mechanisms of tactile working memory. In J. Wu (Ed.), *Biomedical engineering and cognitive neuroscience for healthcare: Interdisciplinary applications* (pp. 89–98). Hershey, PA: IGI Global. doi:10.4018/978-1-4666-2113-8.ch010

Zaheer, S. (2014). Implementation of evidence-based practice and the PARIHS framework. In C. El Morr (Ed.), *Research perspectives on the role of informatics in health policy and management* (pp. 19–36). Hershey, PA: IGI Global. doi:10.4018/978-1-4666-4321-5.ch002

Zalzala, A., Chia, S., Zalzala, L., Sahu, S., Vaghasiya, S., & Karimi, A. (2013). Rural e-health infrastructure development. In I. Management Association (Ed.), User-driven healthcare: Concepts, methodologies, tools, and applications (pp. 870-900). Hershey, PA: IGI Global. doi:10.4018/978-1-4666-2770-3.ch044

Zapirain, B. G., & Zorrilla, A. M. (2013). Independent living support for disabled and elderly people using cell phones. In M. Cruz-Cunha, I. Miranda, & P. Gonçalves (Eds.), *Handbook of research on ICTs for human-centered healthcare and social care services* (pp. 379–397). Hershey, PA: IGI Global. doi:10.4018/978-1-4666-3986-7.ch020

Zgodavová, K., & Bourek, A. (2013). Potential of web based learning in managing for the sustained success of a healthcare organization based on IMPROHEALTH® project. In I. Management Association (Ed.), User-driven healthcare: Concepts, methodologies, tools, and applications (pp. 1523-1540). Hershey, PA: IGI Global. doi:10.4018/978-1-4666-2770-3.ch076

Zhao, X., Zuo, M. J., & Moghaddass, R. (2013). Generating indicators for diagnosis of fault levels by integrating information from two or more sensors. In I. Management Association (Ed.), User-driven healthcare: Concepts, methodologies, tools, and applications (pp. 288-309). Hershey, PA: IGI Global. doi:10.4018/978-1-4666-2770-3.ch015

Zhou, X., & Ren, X. (2013). Speed-accuracy tradeoff models of target-based and trajectory-based movements. In J. Wu (Ed.), *Biomedical engineering and cognitive neuroscience for healthcare: Interdisciplinary applications* (pp. 355–368). Hershey, PA: IGI Global. doi:10.4018/978-1-4666-2113-8.ch037

Zouag, N., & Driouchi, A. (2014). Trends and prospects of the Moroccan health system: 2010-2030. In A. Driouchi (Ed.), *Labor and health economics in the mediterranean region: Migration and mobility of medical doctors* (pp. 314–336). Hershey, PA: IGI Global. doi:10.4018/978-1-4666-4723-7.ch013

Zvikhachevskaya, A., & Mihaylova, L. (2013). Advanced video distribution for wireless e-healthcare systems. In I. Management Association (Ed.), User-driven healthcare: Concepts, methodologies, tools, and applications (pp. 421-446). Hershey, PA: IGI Global. doi:10.4018/978-1-4666-2770-3.ch021

# Compilation of References

Adibi, S. (Ed.). (2015). *Mobile health: a technology road map* (Vol. 5). Springer.

AES. (n.d.). Retrieved from https://engineering.purdue.edu/kak/compsec / NewLectures/Lecture8.pdf

Aitken, M., & Gauntlett, C. (2013). *Patient apps for improved healthcare: from novelty to mainstream.* Parsippany, NJ: IMS Institute for Healthcare Informatics.

Al-Ayyoub, M., Jararweh, Y., Lo'ai, A., Tawalbeh, E., Benkhelifa & Basalamah. (2015). Power Optimization of Large Scale Mobile Cloud Computing Systems. In *Proceedings of the 3rd IEEE International conference on Future Internet of things and Cloud (Fi- Cloud).* Rome, Italy: IEEE.

Alterovitz, G., Warner, J., Zhang, P., Chen, Y., Ullman-Cullere, M., Kreda, D., & Kohane, I. S. (2015). SMART on FHIR Genomics: Facilitating standardized clinico-genomic apps. *Journal of the American Medical Informatics Association*, 1–6. PMID:26198304

Altowaijri, S., Mehmood, R., & Williams, J. (2010, January). A quantitative model of grid systems performance in healthcare organisations. In *Intelligent Systems, Modelling and Simulation (ISMS), 2010 International Conference on* (pp. 431-436). IEEE. 10.1109/ISMS.2010.84

Altunkan, S., Yasemin, A., Aykac, I., & Akpinar, E. (2012). Turkish pharmaceuticals track amp; trace system. *7th International Symposium on in Health Informatics and Bioinformatics (HIBIT), 2012*, 24-30.

Ando, T., Tsukahara, R., Seki, M., & Fujie, M. G. (2012). A haptic interface "Force blinker 2" for navigation of the visually impaired. *IEEE Transactions on Industrial Electronics, 59*(11), 4112–4119. doi:10.1109/TIE.2011.2173894

Ansi, I. (2003). TS 18308 health informatics-requirements for an electronic health record architecture. ISO.

Apple. (2016). *iOS 8 Health*. Retrieved March 17, 2016, from https://www.apple.com/ios/ios8/health/

Armbrust, M., Fox, A., Griffith, R., Joseph, A. D., Katz, R., Konwinski, A., ... Zaharia, M. (2010). A view of cloud computing. *Communications of the ACM, 53*(4), 50–58. doi:10.1145/1721654.1721672

Atzori, Iera, & Morabito. (2010). The Internet of Things: A survey. *Computer Networks, 54,* 2787-2805.

Aungst, T. D. (2013). Medical applications for pharmacists using mobile devices. *The Annals of Pharmacotherapy, 47*(7-8), 1088–1095. doi:10.1345/aph.1S035 PMID:23821609

Bahwaireth. (2016, June). Experimental Comparison of Simulation Tools for Efficient Cloud and Mobile Cloud Computing Applications. *EURASIP Journal on Information Security., 15.* doi:10.118613635-016-0039-y

Barbaro, M., Caboni, A., Cosseddu, P., Mattana, G., & Bonfiglio, A. (2010). Active devices based on organic semiconductors for wearable applications. *IEEE Transactions on Information Technology in Biomedicine, 14*(3), 758–766. doi:10.1109/TITB.2010.2044798 PMID:20371414

Battaglia, F., & Iannizzotto, G. (2012). An open architecture to develop a handheld device for helping visually impaired people. *IEEE Transactions on Consumer Electronics, 58*(3), 1086–1093. doi:10.1109/TCE.2012.6311360

Bender, D., & Sartipi, K. (2013). HL7 FHIR: An Agile and RESTful approach to healthcare information exchange. In *The 26th IEEE International Symposium on Computer-Based Medical Systems* (pp. 326-331). IEEE.

Benharref, A., & Serhani, M. A. (2014). Novel cloud and SOA-based framework for E-Health monitoring using wireless biosensors. *IEEE Journal of Biomedical and Health Informatics, 18*(1), 46–55. doi:10.1109/JBHI.2013.2262659 PMID:24403403

Benkhelifa, E., Welsh, T., Tawalbeh, L., Khreishah, A., Jararweh, Y., & Al-Ayyoub, M. (2016, March). GA-Based Resource Augmentation Negotation for Energy-Optimised Mobile Ad-hoc Cloud. In *Mobile Cloud Computing, Services, and Engineering (MobileCloud), 2016 4th IEEE International Conference on* (pp. 110-116). IEEE. 10.1109/MobileCloud.2016.25

Benkhelifa, E., Welsh, T., Tawalbeh, L., Jararweh, Y., & Basalamah, A. (2015). User profiling for energy optimisation in mobile cloud computing. *Procedia Computer Science, 52*, 1159–1165. doi:10.1016/j.procs.2015.05.151

Bonato, P. (2005). Advances in wearable technology and applications in physical medicine and rehabilitation. *Journal of Neuroengineering and Rehabilitation, 2*(1), 2. doi:10.1186/1743-0003-2-2 PMID:15733322

Borgia, E. (2014). The Internet of Thigs vision: Key features, application and open issues. *Computer Communications, 54*, 131. doi:10.1016/j.comcom.2014.09.008

Boric-Lubecke, O., Xiaomeng, G., Yavari, E., Baboli, M., Singh, A., & Lubecke, V. M. (2014). E-healthcare: Remote monitoring, privacy, and security. *Microwave Symposium (IMS), 2014 IEEE MTT-S International*, 1-3. 10.1109/MWSYM.2014.6848602

Borodin, A., Zavyalova, Y., Zaharov, A., & Yamushev, I. (2015, April). Architectural approach to the multisource health monitoring application design. In *Open Innovations Association (FRUCT), 2015 17th Conference of* (pp. 16-21). IEEE. 10.1109/FRUCT.2015.7117965

Boukerche, A., & Ren, Y. (2009). A secure mobile healthcare system using trust-based multicast scheme. *IEEE Journal on Selected Areas in Communications, 27*(4), 387–399. doi:10.1109/JSAC.2009.090504

Boulos, M. N. K., Wheeler, S., Tavares, C., & Jones, R. (2011). How smartphones are changing the face of mobile and participatory healthcare: An overview, with an example from eCAALYX. *Biomedical Engineering Online, 10*(1), 1. doi:10.1186/1475-925X-10-24 PMID:21466669

Boyd, R. (2012). *Getting started with OAuth 2.0*. O'Reilly Media, Inc.

Boyi, X., Li Da, X., Hongming, C., Cheng, X., Jingyuan, H., & Fenglin, B. (2014). Ubiquitous Data Accessing Method in IoT-Based Information System for Emergency Medical Services. *Industrial Informatics, IEEE Transactions on, 10*(2), 1578–1586. doi:10.1109/TII.2014.2306382

Catarinucci, L., De Donno, D., Mainetti, L., Palano, L., Patrono, L., Stefanizzi, M. L., & Tarricone, L. (2015). An IoT-Aware Architecture for Smart Healthcare Systems. *Internet of Things Journal, IEEE, 2*(6), 515–526. doi:10.1109/JIOT.2015.2417684

Chakravorty, R. (2006). MobiCare: A programmable service architecture for mobile medical care. In *Fourth Annual IEEE International Conference on Pervasive Computing and Communications Workshops (PERCOMW'06)* (pp. 5). IEEE.

Chiuchisan, I., Chiuchisan, I., & Dimian, M. (2015, October). Internet of Things for e-Health: An approach to medical applications. In *Computational Intelligence for Multimedia Understanding (IWCIM), 2015 International Workshop on* (pp. 1-5). IEEE.

Chung, Lee, & Toh. (2008). WSN based mobile u-healthcare system with ECG, blood pressure measurement function. *30th Annual International Conference of the IEEE, Engineering in Medicine and Biology Society*, 1533 – 1536.

Council, C. S. C. (2012). *Impact of cloud computing on healthcare. Technical report*. Cloud Standards Customer Council.

CVS Pharmacy. (2016). *CVS mHealth*. Retrieved February 13, 2016, from http://www.cvs.com/mobile-cvs

Darwish, A., & Hassanien, A. E. (2011). Wearable and implantable wireless sensor network solutions for healthcare monitoring. *Sensors (Basel), 11*(6), 5561–5595. doi:10.3390110605561 PMID:22163914

Data Protection for the Healthcare Industry. (n.d.). Retrieved from http://www.safenet-inc.com/uploadedF iles/About_SafeNet/Resource_Library/Resource_Items/White_PapersSFDC_Protected_EDP/SafeNet%20Data%20Protection%20Healthcare%20White%20Paper.pdf

Delmastro, F. (2012). Pervasive communications in healthcare. *Computer Communications, 35*(11), 1284–1295. doi:10.1016/j.comcom.2012.04.018

Deshmukh, S. D., & Shilaskar, S. N. (2015, January). Wearable sensors and patient monitoring system: A Review. In *Pervasive Computing (ICPC), 2015 International Conference on* (pp. 1-3). IEEE. 10.1109/PERVASIVE.2015.7086982

Drugs.com. (2016). *Drugs.com mHealth*. Retrieved March 19, 2016, from http://www.drugs.com/apps/

Dudde, R., Vering, T., Piechotta, G., & Hintsche, R. (2006). Computer-aided continuous drug infusion: Setup and test of a mobile closed-loop system for the continuous automated infusion of insulin. *IEEE Transactions on Information Technology in Biomedicine, 10*(2), 395–402. doi:10.1109/TITB.2006.864477 PMID:16617628

Evans, D. (2011). The internet of things: How the next evolution of the internet is changing everything. *CISCO White Paper, 1*(2011), 1-11.

Fielding, R. T. (2000). *Architectural styles and the design of network-based software architectures* (Doctoral dissertation). Irvine, CA: University of California.

Fox, A., Griffith, R., Joseph, A., Katz, R., Konwinski, A., Lee, G., . . . Stoica, I. (2009). Above the clouds: A Berkeley view of cloud computing. Dept. Electrical Eng. and Comput. Sciences, University of California, Berkeley, Rep. UCB/EECS, 28(13), 2009.

Franz, B., Schuler, A., & Kraus, O. (2015). *Applying FHIR in an Integrated Health Monitoring System*. EJBI.

Funt, S. (2016). *My Imaging Records App*. Retrieved March 22, 2016, from http://myimagingrecords.com/index.html

Google. (2016). *Fitness Tracker App*. Retrieved March 15, 2016, from https://play.google.com/store/apps/details?id=com.realitinc.fitnesstracker

Gope, P., & Hwang, T. (2016). BSN-Care: A secure IoT-based modern healthcare system using body sensor network. *IEEE Sensors Journal, 16*(5), 1368–1376. doi:10.1109/JSEN.2015.2502401

Goswami. (2013). Mobile Computing. *Int. J. Adv. Res. Comput. Sci. Softw. Eng.*, 846–855.

Guo, Y., Kuo, M. H., & Sahama, T. (2012, December). Cloud computing for healthcare research information sharing. In *Cloud Computing Technology and Science (CloudCom), 2012 IEEE 4th International Conference on* (pp. 889-894). IEEE. 10.1109/CloudCom.2012.6427561

Gupta, M. S. D., Patchava, V., & Menezes, V. (2015, October). Healthcare based on IoT using Raspberry Pi. In *Green Computing and Internet of Things (ICGCIoT), 2015 International Conference on* (pp. 796-799). IEEE. 10.1109/ICGCIoT.2015.7380571

HAPI Community. (2016). *About HAPI.* Retrieved March 23, 2016, from http://hl7api.sourceforge.net/

Health Level 7. (2016a). *About HL7.* Retrieved March 14, 2016, from http://www.hl7.org/

Health Level 7. (2016b). *Clinical Document Architecture.* Retrieved March 15, 2016, from http://www.hl7.org/implement/standards/product_brief. cfm?product_id=7

Health Level 7. (2016c). *Fast Health Interoperable Resources.* Retrieved March 16, 2016, from http://www.hl7.org/implement/standards/fhir/

Health Level 7. (2016d). *Health Intersections FHIR Server.* Retrieved March 08, 2016, from http://fhir2.healthintersections.com.au/open

Health Level 7. (2016e). *HL7 Version 2.* Retrieved March 14, 2016, from http://www.hl7.org/implement/standards/product_brief.cfm?product_id=185

Health Level 7. (2016f). *HL7 Version 3.* Retrieved March 14, 2016, from https://www.hl7.org/implement/standards/product_brief.cfm?product_id=186

Health Relationship Trust Working Group. (2016). *HEART profile for FHIR.* Retrieved March 22, 2016, from http://openid.net/wg/heart/

Henneman, E. A., Gawlinski, A., & Giuliano, K. K. (2012). Surveillance: A strategy for improving patient safety in acute and critical care units. *Critical Care Nurse, 32*(2), e9–e18. doi:10.4037/ccn2012166 PMID:22467622

Huang, D., & ... (2011). Mobile cloud computing. *IEEE COMSOC Multimed. Commun. Tech. Comm. MMTC E-Lett., 6*(10), 27–31.

Hussain, M. I. (2017). Internet of Things: challenges and research opportunities. *CSI Transactions on ICT, 5*(1), 87-95.

IBM. (2011). *Cloud Computing: Building a New Foundation for Healthcare.* IBM Corporation. Available: https://www-05.ibm.com/de/healthcare/literature/cloud-newfoundation- for-hv.pdf

ITU-T Technology watch report. (2013). *Smart cities Seoul: A case study.* Author.

Jadhav, P., Devkatte, B., & Dhumal, V. (2015). The health care monitoring using android mobile phone. *IJETT, 2*(1).

James, J. T. (2013). A new, evidence-based estimate of patient harms associated with hospital care. *Journal of Patient Safety*, *9*(3), 122–128. doi:10.1097/PTS.0b013e3182948a69 PMID:23860193

Jararweh, Y., Ababneh, F., Khreishah, A., & Dosari, F. (2014). Scalable cloudlet-based mobile computing model. *Procedia Computer Science*, *34*, 434–441. doi:10.1016/j.procs.2014.07.051

Jethjarurach, N., & Limpiyakorn, Y. (2014). Mobile Product Barcode Reader for Thai Blinds. *International Conference on Information Science and Applications (ICISA)*, 1-4. 10.1109/ICISA.2014.6847426

José, J., Farrajota, M., Rodrigues, J. M., & Du Buf, J. H. (2011). The SmartVision local navigation aid for blind and visually impaired persons. *International Journal of Digital Content Technology and its Applications*, *5*(5), 362-375.

Joseph, S. L., Xiao, J., Chawda, B., Narang, K., & Janarthanam, P. (2014, June). A blind user-centered navigation system with crowdsourced situation awareness. In *Cyber Technology in Automation, Control, and Intelligent Systems (CYBER), 2014 IEEE 4th Annual International Conference on* (pp. 186-191). IEEE. 10.1109/CYBER.2014.6917458

Jovanov, E., Milenkovic, A., Otto, C., & De Groen, P. C. (2005). A wireless body area network of intelligent motion sensors for computer assisted physical rehabilitation. *Journal of Neuroengineering and Rehabilitation*, *2*(1), 6. doi:10.1186/1743-0003-2-6 PMID:15740621

Jubadi, W. M., & Sahak, S. F. A. M. (2009, October). Heartbeat monitoring alert via SMS. In *Industrial Electronics & Applications, 2009. ISIEA 2009. IEEE Symposium on* (Vol. 1, pp. 1-5). IEEE. 10.1109/ISIEA.2009.5356491

Kahanwal, Dua, & Singh. (2012). Java File Security System. *Global Journal of Computer Science and Technology Network and Web Security, 12*(10).

Kailash, M., Manokar, P., & Manokar, N. V. (2013). Scanmedic through e-governance. *7th International Conference on Intelligent Systems and Control (ISCO)*, 480-483.

Kale, A. V., Gawade, S. D., Jadhav, S. Y., & Patil, S. A. (2015). GSM Based Heart Rate and Temperature Monitoring System. *International Journal of Engineering Research & Technology, 4*(4).

Kasthurirathne, S. N., Mamlin, B., Kumara, H., Grieve, G., & Biondich, P. (2015). Enabling Better Interoperability for HealthCare: Lessons in Developing a Standards Based Application Programing Interface for Electronic Medical Record Systems. *Journal of Medical Systems*, 1–8. PMID:26446013

Kay, M., Santos, J., & Takane, M. (2011). mHealth: New horizons for health through mobile technologies. *World Health Organization, 64*(7), 66-71.

Khemapech. (2005). *A Survey of Wireless Sensor Net-works Technology. In 6th Annual Postgraduate Symposium on the Convergence of Telecommunications, Networking and Broadcasting.* Liverpool, UK: Liverpool John Moores University.

Kim, J. E., Bessho, M., Koshizuka, N., & Sakamura, K. (2014, December). Mobile applications for assisting mobility for the visually impaired using IoT infrastructure. In *TRON Symposium (TRONSHOW)*, 2014 (pp. 1-6). IEEE.

Kohn, L. T., Corrigan, J. M., & Donaldson, M. S. (Eds.). (2000). *To err is human: building a safer health system* (Vol. 6). National Academies Press.

Kumar, P., & Lee, H. J. (2011). Security issues in healthcare applications using wireless medical sensor networks: A survey. *Sensors (Basel), 12*(1), 55–91. doi:10.3390120100055 PMID:22368458

La, H. J., Kim, M. K., & Kim, S. D. (2015, June). A Personal Healthcare System with Inference-as-a-Service. In *Services Computing (SCC), 2015 IEEE International Conference on* (pp. 249-255). IEEE. 10.1109/SCC.2015.42

Lamprinakos, G. C., Mousas, A. S., Kapsalis, A. P., Kaklamani, D. I., Venieris, I. S., Boufis, A. D., & Mantzouratos, S. G. (2014). *Using FHIR to develop a healthcare mobile application. In Wireless Mobile Communication and Healthcare (Mobihealth)* (pp. 132–135). IEEE.

Lanatà, A., Scilingo, E. P., Nardini, E., Loriga, G., Paradiso, R., & De-Rossi, D. (2010). Comparative evaluation of susceptibility to motion artifact in different wearable systems for monitoring respiratory rate. *IEEE Transactions on Information Technology in Biomedicine, 14*(2), 378–386. doi:10.1109/TITB.2009.2037614 PMID:20007035

Lin, S.-C., & Wang, P.-H. (2014). Design of a barcode identification system. *IEEE International Conference on Consumer Electronics - Taiwan (ICCE-TW),* 237-238. 10.1109/ICCE-TW.2014.6904077

Lin, C. C., Chiu, M. J., Hsiao, C. C., Lee, R. G., & Tsai, Y. S. (2006). Wireless health care service system for elderly with dementia. *IEEE Transactions on Information Technology in Biomedicine, 10*(4), 696–704. doi:10.1109/TITB.2006.874196 PMID:17044403

Lo'ai, A. T., & Bakhader, W. (2016, August). A Mobile Cloud System for Different Useful Applications. In *Future Internet of Things and Cloud Workshops (FiCloudW), IEEE International Conference on* (pp. 295-298). IEEE.

Lo'ai, A. T., Bakheder, W., & Song, H. (2016, June). A mobile cloud computing model using the cloudlet scheme for big data applications. In *Connected Health: Applications, Systems and Engineering Technologies (CHASE), 2016 IEEE First International Conference on* (pp. 73-77). IEEE.

Lo'ai, A. T., Bakhader, W., Mehmood, R., & Song, H. (2016, December). Cloudlet-based Mobile Cloud Computing for Healthcare Applications. In *Global Communications Conference (GLOBECOM)* (pp. 1-6). IEEE.

Lo, B., & Yang, G. Z. (2005, April). Key technical challenges and current implementations of body sensor networks. *Proc. 2nd International Workshop on Body Sensor Networks (BSN 2005)*.

Loomis, J. M., Marston, J. R., Golledge, R. G., & Klatzky, R. L. (2005). Personal guidance system for people with visual impairment: A comparison of spatial displays for route guidance. *Journal of Visual Impairment & Blindness, 99*(4), 219. PMID:20054426

Macias, F., & Thomas, G. (2011). *Cloud Computing Advantages in the Public Sector: How Today's Government, Education, and Healthcare Organizations Are Benefiting from Cloud Computing Environments*. Retrieved from Cisco website: http://www. cisco. com/web/strategy/docs/c11-687784_cloud_omputing_wp. pdf

Makary, M. A., & Daniel, M. (2016). Medical error—the third leading cause of death in the US. *BMJ (Clinical Research Ed.), 353*, i2139. PMID:27143499

Mandel, J. C., Kreda, D. A., Mandl, K. D., Kohane, I. S., & Ramoni, R. B. (2016). SMART on FHIR: a standards-based, interoperable apps platform for electronic health records. *Journal of the American Medical Informatics Association*. Retrieved March 25, 2016, from http://docs.smarthealthit.org/

Manjula. (n.d.). *Lab manual on mobile application development lab*. Dept of Information Technology, Institute of Aeronautical Engineering Dundigal.

Marsh, A., May, M., & Saarelainen, M. (2000). Pharos: coupling GSM and GPS-TALK technologies to provide orientation, navigation and location-based services for the blind. In *Information Technology Applications in Biomedicine, 2000. Proceedings. 2000 IEEE EMBS International Conference on* (pp. 38-43). IEEE. 10.1109/ITAB.2000.892345

Mazidi, M. A., McKinlay, R. D., & Causey, D. (2008). *PIC microcontroller and embedded systems: using Assembly and C for PIC18*. Academic Press.

MEDWATCHER. (2016). *MEDWATCHER mHealth*. Retrieved March 18, 2016, from https://medwatcher.org/

Mehmood, R., Faisal, M. A., & Altowaijri, S. (n.d.). Future Networked Healthcare Systems: A Review and Case Study. In Handbook Res. Redesigning Future Internet Archit. (pp. 564–590). Academic Press.

Mehmood, R., & Graham, G. (2015). Big data logistics: A health-care transport capacity sharing model. *Procedia Computer Science, 64*, 1107–1114. doi:10.1016/j.procs.2015.08.566

Mell, P., & Grance, T. (2010). *The NIST definition of cloud computing*. NIST.

Mickan, S., Tilson, J. K., Atherton, H., Roberts, N. W., & Heneghan, C. (2013). Evidence of effectiveness of health care professionals using handheld computers: A scoping review of systematic reviews. *Journal of Medical Internet Research, 15*(10), 212. doi:10.2196/jmir.2530 PMID:24165786

Middleton, N., & Schneeman, R. (2013). *Heroku: Up and Running*. O'Reilly Media, Inc.

Miettinen, A. P., & Nurminen, J. K. (2010). Energy Efficiency of Mobile Clients in Cloud Computing. *HotCloud, 10*, 4–4.

Milenković, A., Otto, C., & Jovanov, E. (2006). Wireless sensor networks for personal health monitoring: Issues and an implementation. *Computer Communications, 29*(13), 2521–2533. doi:10.1016/j.comcom.2006.02.011

Moh'd, A., Aslam, N., Marzi, H., & Tawalbeh, L. A. (2010, July). Hardware implementations of secure hashing functions on FPGAs for WSNs. *Proceedings of the 3rd International Conference on the Applications of Digital Information and Web Technologies (ICADIWT.*

Mohammad, A., & Gutub, A. A. A. (2010). Efficient FPGA implementation of a programmable architecture for GF (p) elliptic curve crypto computations. *Journal of Signal Processing Systems for Signal, Image, and Video Technology, 59*(3), 233–244. doi:10.1007/11265-009-0376-x

Moore, S. (2015). *Gartner Says Demand for Enterprise Mobile Apps Will Outstrip Available Development Capacity Five to One*. Retrieved March 13, 2016, from http://www.gartner.com/newsroom/id/3076817

Moorthi, M. N., & Vaideeswaran, J. (n.d.). *Design of an Embedded System for Health Monitoring and Emergency services using wearable sensors*. Academic Press.

Morris, D., Schazmann, B., Wu, Y., Coyle, S., Brady, S., Fay, C., . . . Diamond, D. (2008, August). Wearable technology for bio-chemical analysis of body fluids during exercise. In *Engineering in Medicine and Biology Society, 2008. EMBS 2008. 30th Annual International Conference of the IEEE* (pp. 5741-5744). IEEE. 10.1109/IEMBS.2008.4650518

Mosa, A. S. M., Yoo, I., & Sheets, L. (2012). A systematic review of healthcare applications for smartphones. *BMC Medical Informatics and Decision Making, 12*(1), 1. doi:10.1186/1472-6947-12-67 PMID:22781312

MTBC. (2016). *MTBC PHR*. Retrieved March 18, 2016, from https://phr.mtbc.com/

Mulligan, G., & Gra, D. (2009). *A comparison of SOAP and REST implementations of a service based interaction independence middleware framework. In The 2009 Winter Simulation Conference (WSC)* (pp. 1423–1432). IEEE.

Narayana Moorthi & Manjula. (n.d.). Developing a framework for automated patient care monitoring system for medical clinics using 8051 microcontroller. *IJPBS*.

Natarajan, K., Prasath, B., & Kokila, P. (2016). Smart health care system using internet of things. *Journal of Network Communications and Emerging Technologies, 6*(3).

Navya, K., & Murthy, M. B. R. (2013). A zigbee based patient health monitoring system. *Int. Journal of Engineering Research and Applications, 3*(5).

Niver, H. M. (2014). *Getting to Know Arduino*. The Rosen Publishing Group.

Nosrati, M., Karimi, R., & Hasanvand, H. A. (2012). Mobile computing: Principles, devices and operating systems. *World Applied Programming, 2*(7), 399–408.

O'Neill, K. M., Holmer, H., Greenberg, S. L., & Meara, J. G. (2013). Applying surgical apps: Smartphone and tablet apps prove useful in clinical practice. *Bulletin of the American College of Surgeons, 98*(11), 10–18. PMID:24313133

OAuth. (2016). *About OAuth 2.0*. Retrieved March 06, 2016, from https://oauth.net/2/

OEMR. (2016). *About OpenEMR*. Retrieved March 11, 2016, from http://www.open-emr.org/

Ohbuchi, E., Hanaizumi, H., & Hock, L. (2004). Barcode readers using the camera device in mobile phones. *International Conference on Cyberworlds*, 260-265. 10.1109/CW.2004.23

Ohsaga, A., & Kondoh, K. (2013). Bedside medication safety management system using a PDA and RFID tags. *7th International Symposium on Medical Information and Communication Technology (ISMICT)*, 85-89. 10.1109/ISMICT.2013.6521705

Ong, S. K., Chai, D., & Rassau, A. (2011). A robust mobile business card reader using MMCC barcode. *IEEE Symposium on Computers Informatics (ISCI)*, 656-661. 10.1109/ISCI.2011.5958994

Open, I. D. (2016). *About OpenID Connect*. Retrieved March 24, 2016, from http://openid.net/connect/

OpenMRS Incorporation. (2016). *About OpenMRS*. Retrieved March 10, 2016, from http://openmrs.org/

Ozdalga, E., Ozdalga, A., & Ahuja, N. (2012). The smartphone in medicine: A review of current and potential use among physicians and students. *Journal of Medical Internet Research, 14*(5), e128. doi:10.2196/jmir.1994 PMID:23017375

Ozkil, A. G., Fan, Z., Dawids, S., Aanes, H., Kristensen, J. K., & Christensen, K. H. (2009, August). Service robots for hospitals: A case study of transportation tasks in a hospital. In *Automation and Logistics, 2009. ICAL'09. IEEE International Conference on* (pp. 289-294). IEEE. 10.1109/ICAL.2009.5262912

Pal, A. (2016). Internet of things making the hype a reality. Innovation Lab, Tata Consultancy Services.

Parvu, O., Balan, A., & Homorogan, A. (2011). A case for online real-time barcode readers. *19th Telecommunications Forum (TELFOR)*, 1546-1549. 10.1109/TELFOR.2011.6143853

Patterson, J. A., McIlwraith, D. C., & Yang, G. Z. (2009, June). A flexible, low noise reflective PPG sensor platform for ear-worn heart rate monitoring. In *Wearable and Implantable Body Sensor Networks, 2009. BSN 2009. Sixth International Workshop on* (pp. 286-291). IEEE. 10.1109/BSN.2009.16

Peng, E., Peursum, P., & Li, L. (2012). Product Barcode and Expiry Date Detection for the Visually Impaired Using a Smartphone. *International Conference on Digital Image Computing Techniques and Applications (DICTA)*, 1-7. 10.1109/DICTA.2012.6411673

Perera, C., Liu, C. H., & Jayawardena, S. (2015) The emerging internet of things marketplace from an industrial perspective: A survey. *IEEE Transactions on Emerging Topics in Computing, 3*(4), 585–598. doi:10.1109/TETC.2015.2390034

Pounraj, P., Winston, D. P., Christabel, S. C., & Ramaraj, R. (2016). A Continuous Health Monitoring System for Photovoltaic Array Using Arduino Microcontroller. *Circuits and Systems, 7*(11), 3494–3503. doi:10.4236/cs.2016.711297

Qi, H., & Gani, A. (2012, May). Research on mobile cloud computing: Review, trend and perspectives. In *Digital Information and Communication Technology and it's Applications (DICTAP), 2012 Second International Conference on* (pp. 195-202). IEEE.

Quest Diagnostics. (2016). *MyQuest Apps*. Retrieved March 20, 2016, from https://myquest.questdiagnostics.com/web/home

Rahmani, A. M., Thanigaivelan, N. K., Gia, T. N., Granados, J., Negash, B., Liljeberg, P., & Tenhunen, H. (2015, January). Smart e-health gateway: Bringing intelligence to internet-of-things based ubiquitous healthcare systems. In *Consumer Communications and Networking Conference (CCNC), 2015 12th Annual IEEE* (pp. 826-834). IEEE. 10.1109/CCNC.2015.7158084

Rajan, Spanias, Ranganath, Banavar, & Spanias. (n.d.). *Health Monitoring Laboratories by Interfacing Physiological Sensors to Mobile Android Devices*. SenSIPCenter, School of ECEE, Arizona State University.

Rajathi, A., & Saravanan, N. (2013). A Survey on Secure Storage in Cloud Computing. *Indian Journal of Science and Technology*, 6(4).

Ren, Y., Werner, R., Pazzi, N., & Boukerche, A. (2010). Monitoring patients via a secure and mobile healthcare system. *IEEE Wireless Communications*, 17(1), 59–65. doi:10.1109/MWC.2010.5416351

Rickwood, S., Kleinrock, M., Núñez-Gaviria, M., & Sakhrani, S. (2013). *The Global Use of Medicines: Outlook through 2017*. Parsippany, NJ: IMS Institute for Healthcare Informatics.

Rivera Sánchez, K. Y., Demurjian, S., Conover, J., Agresta, T., Shao, X., & Diamond, M. (2016). An Approach for Role-Based Access Control in Mobile Applications. In S. Mukherja (Ed.), Mobile Application Development, Usability, and Security. IGI Global.

Rosamond, W., Flegal, K., Friday, G., Furie, K., Go, A., Greenlund, K., ... Hong, Y. (2007). American Heart Association Statistics Committee and Stroke Statistics Subcommittee. Heart disease and stroke statistics-2007 update: A report from the American heart association statistics committee and stroke statistics subcommittee. *Circulation*, 115(5), e69–e171. doi:10.1161/CIRCULATIONAHA.106.179918 PMID:17194875

Seales, C., Do, T., Belyi, E., & Kumar, S. (2015, June). PHINet: A Plug-n-Play Content-centric Testbed Framework for Health-Internet of Things. In *Mobile Services (MS), 2015 IEEE International Conference on* (pp. 368-375). IEEE. 10.1109/MobServ.2015.57

Sebestyen, G., Hangan, A., Oniga, S., & Gal, Z. (2014). eHealth solutions in the context of Internet of Things. *Automation, Quality and Testing, Robotics, 2014 IEEE International Conference*, 1-6. 10.1109/AQTR.2014.6857876

Senate and House of Representatives in General. (2014). *An act concerning youth athletics and concussions*. Hartford, CT: Author.

Serdaroglu, K., Uslu, G., & Baydere, S. (2015, October). Medication intake adherence with real time activity recognition on IoT. In *Wireless and Mobile Computing, Networking and Communications (WiMob), 2015 IEEE 11th International Conference on* (pp. 230-237). IEEE. 10.1109/WiMOB.2015.7347966

Setyowati, V., & Muninggar, J. (2017, January). Design of heart rate monitor based on piezoelectric sensor using an Arduino. *Journal of Physics: Conference Series*, *795*(1), 012016. doi:10.1088/1742-6596/795/1/012016

Shany, T., Redmond, S. J., Narayanan, M. R., & Lovell, N. H. (2012). Sensors-based wearable systems for monitoring of human movement and falls. *IEEE Sensors Journal*, *12*(3), 658–670. doi:10.1109/JSEN.2011.2146246

She, H., Lu, Z., Jantsch, A., Zheng, L. R., & Zhou, D. (2007, August). A network-based system architecture for remote medical applications. In *Network Research Workshop* (*Vol. 27*). Academic Press.

Shiraz, M., & Gani, A. (2012, February). Mobile cloud computing: Critical analysis of application deployment in virtual machines. In *Proc. Int'l Conf. Information and Computer Networks (ICICN'12)* (*Vol. 27*). Academic Press.

Silva, B. M., Lopes, I. M., Marques, M. B., Rodrigues, J. J., & Proença, M. L. (2013). A mobile health application for outpatient's medication management. In *2013 IEEE International Conference on Communications (ICC)* (pp. 4389-4393). IEEE. 10.1109/ICC.2013.6655256

Smith, A. (2015). *U.S. Smartphone Use in 2015*. Retrieved January 08, 2016, from http://www.pewinternet.org/2015/04/01/us-smartphone-use-in-2015/

Son, D., Lee, J., Qiao, S., Ghaffari, R., Kim, J., Lee, J. E., ... Yang, S. (2014). Multifunctional wearable devices for diagnosis and therapy of movement disorders. *Nature Nanotechnology*, *9*(5), 397–404. doi:10.1038/nnano.2014.38 PMID:24681776

Spencer, B. F. Jr, Ruiz-Sandoval, M., & Kurata, N. (2004, August). Smart sensing technology for structural health monitoring. *Proceedings of the 13th World Conference on Earthquake Engineering*.

Sreekanth, K. U., & Nitha, K. P. (2016). A study on health Care in Internet of Things. *International Journal on Recent and Innovation Trends in Computing and Communication*, *4*(2), 44–47.

Stankevich, E., Paramonov, I., & Timofeev, I. (2012, April). Mobile phone sensors in health applications. In *Proc. 12th Conf. of Open Innovations Association FRUCT and Seminar on e-Tourism* (pp. 136-141). Academic Press.

Strisland, F., Svagard, I., & Seeberg, T.M. (2013). ESUMS: A mobile system for continuous home monitoring of rehabilitation patient. *Proceedings of the 35th IEEE Annual International Conference on Engineering in Medicine and Biology Society*, 4670-4673.

Suhair, A. B., Golisano, T., Radziszowski, S. P., & Raj, R. K. (2012). Secure Access for Healthcare Data in the Cloud Using cipher text-Policy Attribute-Based Encryption. *Proc of International Conference on Data Engineering Workshop.*

Sundaram, P. (2013). Patient monitoring system using android technology. *International Journal of Computer Science and Mobile Computing, 2*(5), 191–201.

Suryadevara, N. K., & Mukhopadhyay, S. C. (2012). Wireless sensor network based home monitoring system for wellness determination of elderly. *IEEE Sensors Journal, 12*(6), 1965–1972. doi:10.1109/JSEN.2011.2182341

Tang, L. Z. W., Ang, K. S., Amirul, M., Yusoff, M. B. M., Tng, C. K., Alyas, M. D. B. M., . . . Folianto, F. (2015, April). Augmented reality control home (ARCH) for disabled and elderlies. In *Intelligent Sensors, Sensor Networks and Information Processing (ISSNIP), 2015 IEEE Tenth International Conference on* (pp. 1-2). IEEE.

Tartarisco, G., Baldus, G., Corda, D., Raso, R., Arnao, A., Ferro, M., ... Pioggia, G. (2012). Personal Health System architecture for stress monitoring and support to clinical decisions. *Computer Communications, 35*(11), 1296–1305. doi:10.1016/j.comcom.2011.11.015

Tawalbeh, L. A., Alassaf, N., Bakheder, W., & Tawalbeh, A. (2015, October). Resilience Mobile Cloud Computing: Features, Applications and Challenges. In *e-Learning (econf), 2015 Fifth International Conference on* (pp. 280-284). IEEE.

Tawalbeh, L. A., Jararweh, Y., & Mohammad, A. (2012). An integrated radix-4 modular divider/multiplier hardware architecture for cryptographic applications. *The International Arab Journal of Information Technology, 9*(3).

Tawalbeh, L. A., Tenca, A. F., Park, S., & Koc, C. K. (2004). A dualfield modular division algorithm and architecture for application specific hardware. In *Thirty-Eighth Asilomar Conference on Signals, Systems, and Computers* (pp. 483-487). IEEE Press.

Tawalbeh, M., Eardley, A., & Tawalbeh, L. (2016). Studying the energy consumption in mobile devices. *Procedia Computer Science*, *94*, 183–189. doi:10.1016/j.procs.2016.08.028

Touati, F., & Tabish, R. (2013). Towards u-health: An indoor 6LoWPAN based platform for real-time healthcare monitoring. *Proceedings of the IFIP International Conference on Wireless and Mobile Networking*, 1-4.

Ufoaroh, S. U., Oranugo, C. O., & Uchechukwu, M. E. (2015). Heartbeat monitoring and alert system using GSM technology. *International Journal of Engineering Research and General Science*, *3*(4), 26–34.

University of California San Francisco Library. (2016). *Mobile Apps for Healthcare Professionals*. Retrieved January 19, 2016, from http://guides.ucsf.edu/c.php?g=100993&p=654826

Valentin, A., Capuzzo, M., Guidet, B., Moreno, R. P., Dolanski, L., Bauer, P., & Metnitz, P. G. (2006). Patient safety in intensive care: Results from the multinational Sentinel Events Evaluation (SEE) study. *Intensive Care Medicine*, *32*(10), 1591–1598. doi:10.100700134-006-0290-7 PMID:16874492

Varshney, U. (2007). Pervasive healthcare and wireless health monitoring. *Mobile Networks and Applications*, *12*(2-3), 113–127. doi:10.100711036-007-0017-1

Wakita, K., Huang, J., Di, P., Sekiyama, K., & Fukuda, T. (2013). Human-walking-intention-based motion control of an omnidirectional-type cane robot. *IEEE/ASME Transactions on Mechatronics*, *18*(1), 285–296. doi:10.1109/TMECH.2011.2169980

Walker, J., Pan, E., Johnston, D., & Adler-Milstein, J. (2005). The value of health care information exchange and interoperability. *Health Affairs*, *24*. PMID:15659453

Wang, M. Y., Tsai, P. H., Liu, J. W. S., & Zao, J. K. (2009). Wedjat: a mobile phone based medicine intake reminder and monitor. In *Bioinformatics and BioEngineering, 2009. BIBE'09. Ninth IEEE International Conference on.* (pp. 423-430). IEEE.

Wang, L., Yang, G. Z., Huang, J., Zhang, J., Yu, L., Nie, Z., & Cumming, D. R. S. (2010). A wireless biomedical signal interface system-on-chip for body sensor networks. *IEEE Transactions on Biomedical Circuits and Systems*, *4*(2), 112–117. doi:10.1109/TBCAS.2009.2038228 PMID:23853318

Web, M. D. (2016). *WebMD Apps*. Retrieved March 12, 2016, from http://www.webmd.com/mobile

Webahn Incorporation. (2016). *Single App to Track Health and Wellness of Your Family*. Retrieved March 19, 2016, from https://www.capzule.com/

Wei, Z., Chaowei, W., & Nakahira, Y. (2011). Medical application on internet of things. *Communication Technology and Application (ICCTA 2011), IET International Conference on*, 660-665.

Weihua, W., Jiangong, L., Ling, W., & Wendong, Z. (2011). The internet of things for resident health information service platform research. *Communication Technology and Application (ICCTA 2011), IET International Conference on*, 631-635. 10.1049/cp.2011.0745

What is Geolocation and How Does it Apply to Network Detection? (n.d.). Retrieved from https://www.sans.org/security-resources/idfaq/what-is-geolocation-and-how-does-it-apply-to-network-detection/1/28

Wood, L. B., & Asada, H. H. (2007, August). Low variance adaptive filter for cancelling motion artifact in wearable photoplethysmogram sensor signals. In *Engineering in Medicine and Biology Society, 2007. EMBS 2007. 29th Annual International Conference of the IEEE* (pp. 652-655). IEEE. 10.1109/IEMBS.2007.4352374

Xu, Xu, Cai, Xie, Hu, & Bu. (2014). Ubiquitous Data Accessing Method in IoT-Based Information System for Emergency Medical Services. *IEEE Transactions on Industrial Informatics*, *10*(2).

Yan, Y. S., & Zhang, Y. T. (2008). An efficient motion-resistant method for wearable pulse oximeter. *IEEE Transactions on Information Technology in Biomedicine*, *12*(3), 399–405. doi:10.1109/TITB.2007.902173 PMID:18693507

Yuan Jie, F., Yue Hong, Y., Li Da, X., Yan, Z., & Fan, W. (2014). IoT-Based Smart Rehabilitation System. *Industrial Informatics, IEEE Transactions on*, *10*(2), 1568–157. doi:10.1109/TII.2014.2302583

Zanella, A., Bui, N., Castellani, A., Vangelista, L., & Zorzi, M. (2014). Internet of things for smart cities. *IEEE Internet of Things Journal*, *1*(1), 22-32.

Zao, J. K., Wang, M. Y., Tsai, P., & Liu, J. W. (2010). Smartphone based medicine intake scheduler, reminder, and monitor. In *e-Health Networking Applications and Services (Healthcom), 2010 12th IEEE International Conference on*. (pp. 162-168). IEEE.

Zhao, Y. J., Davidson, A., Bain, J., Li, S. Q., Wang, Q., & Lin, Q. (2005, June). A MEMS viscometric glucose monitoring device. In *Solid-State Sensors, Actuators and Microsystems, 2005. Digest of Technical Papers. TRANSDUCERS'05. The 13th International Conference on* (Vol. 2, pp. 1816-1819). IEEE. 10.1109/SENSOR.2005.1497447

Zimmerman, J. B. (1999). Mobile computing: Characteristics, business benefits, and the mobile framework. *University of Maryland European Division-Bowie State*, *10*, 12.

# About the Contributors

**R. Rajkumar** is a Head of the Department and Professor in the School of Computer Science and Engineering at VIT University, India.

\* \* \*

**Thomas Agresta** is Full Professor and Director of Medical Informatics in the Department of Family Medicine at the University of Connecticut Health Center, Director of Clinical Informatics for the Biomedical Informatics Division of the Center for Quantitative Medicine, and is the Section Leader for Informatics at the Connecticut Institute for Primary Care Innovation. He is a family physician with more than 25 years of experience caring for patients at Asylum Hill Family Medicine Center in Hartford, CT. He is Board Certified in Clinical Informatics and is nationally known for his innovative approach to teaching students, residents and physicians to use technology at point of care to provide patient-centered, evidence-based care.

**Mohammed S. Baihan** is a Ph.D. student at the Computer Science & Engineering department at the University of Connecticut. His research interests include developing a security infrastructure that is needed to support the secure access control (via RBAC, DAC, and/or MAC) of mobile applications that are built using cloud computing services.

**S. A. Demurjian** is a Full Professor in Computer Science & Engineering at the University of Connecticut, and co-Director of Research Informatics for the Biomedical Informatics Division, with research interests of: secure-software engineering, security for biomedical applications, and security-web architectures. Dr. Demurjian has over 160 archival publications, in the following categories: 1 book, 2 edited collections, 65 journal articles and book chapters, and 99 refereed conference/workshop articles.

**C. Gilman** is a Research Associate in the Computer Science & Engineering department at the University of Connecticut in charge of various systems and technologies in support of biomedical informatics at UConn including FHIR, OpenEMR, and OpenMRS.

**Govinda K.** is an Associate Professor in School of Computing Science and Engineering and area of interest include Database, Data Mining, Cloud Computing and IOT.

**Narayana Moorthi M.** is currently working in VIT University, Vellore-14 as Assistant Professor (SG).

**Nalini Nagendhiran** received her M.Sc in Computer Science and M.Tech in Computer Science and Engineering from VIT University, Vellore, India. She is currently with the School of Computer Science and Engineering, VIT University, Vellore, India. She is pursuing her Ph.D with the School of Computer Science and Engineering, VIT University, Vellore, India. She has authored a few research papers in reputed journals. Her research interests are Data Mining, IoT, Mobile and Wireless System.

**Y. K. Rivera Sánchez** is a Ph.D. student at the Computer Science & Engineering department at the University of Connecticut. Her research interests include security for mobile applications, specifically in the authentication and authorization process of them (allow mobile applications to access, share, and exchange information from different sources/applications) and emphasizing on solutions that are suitable for applications in the biomedical and healthcare domains.

**X. Shao** is a Ph.D. student at the Computer Science & Engineering department at the University of Connecticut. Her research interests include security for mobile applications, specifically to allow mobile applications on mobile devices to dynamically adjust permissions based on both the system being utilized and the actual location of the user/device.

**H. Parveen Sultana** received the MCA from Madras University, Chennai, India, and M.Phil in Computer Applications from Manonmaniam Sundaranar University, Tirunelveli, India. She is currently with the School of Computer Science and Engineering, VIT University, Vellore, India. She received her Ph.D from the School of Computer Science and Engineering, VIT University, Vellore, India. Her research interests include Cyber physical systems, mobile and wireless systems and data structures. She has authored a few research papers in various reputed journals and conferences. She also co-authored a book on Cyber Physical Systems.

# Index

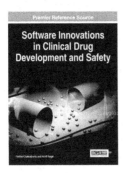
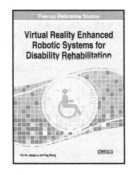
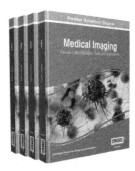
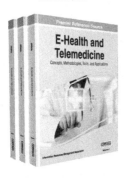
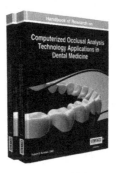
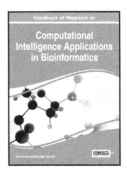
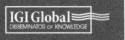

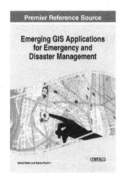
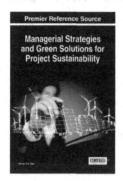
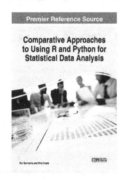
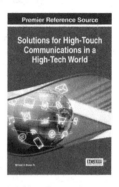

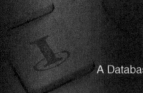
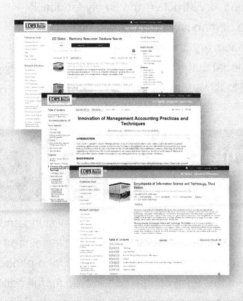
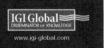

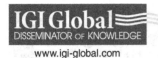
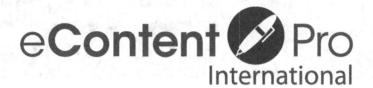
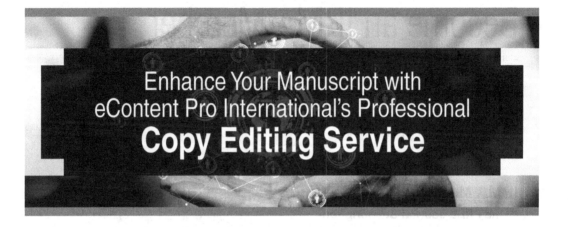

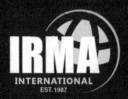
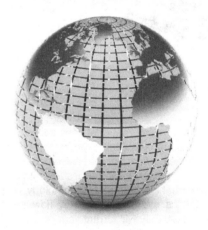

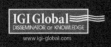
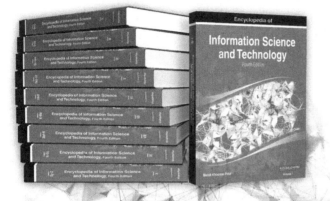